HOPE AND DESTINY

The Adult Patient and
Parent's Guide to
Sickle Cell Disease
and Sickle Cell Trait

· Revised Fifth Edition ·

Allan F. Platt, PA-C, MMSc,
James Eckman, MD, and
Lewis L. Hsu, MD, PhD

Hilton Publishing Company · Chicago, Illinois

Hilton Publishing Company
5261-A Fountain Drive
Crown Point, IN 46307
219-922-4868
www.hiltonpub.com

Fifth edition © 2019 by Allan F. Platt Jr., James Eckman, and Lewis L. Hsu
ISBN-13: 978-0-9983282-5-6
ISBN-10: 0-9983282-5-1

Notice: The information in this book is true and complete to the best of the authors' and publisher's knowledge. This book is intended only as an information reference and should not replace, countermand, or conflict with the advice given to readers by their physicians. The authors and publisher disclaim all liability in connection with the specific personal use of any and all information provided in this book.

All rights reserved. No part of this book may be reproduced or transmitted in any form or by any means, electronic or mechanical, including photocopy, recording, or any information storage or retrieval systems, including digital systems, without written permission from the publisher, except by a reviewer who may quote brief passages from the book in a review.

Map on page 11 used with permission of the World Health Organization.

"Human Body" on page 172 by Tarequl Alam from the Noun Project

Angela Vennemann, Senior Editor and Design
Judine O'Shea, Publisher
Megan Lippert, Executive Vice President, Hilton Publishing Division
Donna Dent, Illustrations

The Library of Congress has cataloged the fourth edition as follows:

Library of Congress Cataloging-In Publication Data

Names: Platt, Allan F., author. | Eckman, James, author. | Hsu, Lewis, author.

Title: Hope and destiny : the patient and parent's guide to sickle cell disease and sickle cell trait / Allan F. Platt, P.A.C, M.M.Sc., James Eckman, M.D., and Lewis Hsu, M.D., Ph.D.

Description: Revised Fourth edition. | Indianapolis, Indiana : Hilton Publishing Company, [2016] | Includes bibliographical references and index.

Identifiers: LCCN 2016026926 (print) | LCCN 2016027817 (ebook) | ISBN 9780984756681 (pbk. : alk. paper) | ISBN 9780984756698 (e-book)

Subjects: LCSH: Sickle cell anemia. | Sickle cell anemia in children.

Classification: LCC RC641.7.S5 P56 2016 (print) | LCC RC641.7.S5 (ebook) | DDC 616.1/527—dc23

LC record available at https://lccn.loc.gov/2016026926

*In memory of
Ingrid Whittaker-Ware, Esq.,
who lived and shared her hopes
and fulfilled her destiny.*

AUTHORS

Allan Platt, PA-C, MMSc, graduated with a BS in Health Systems Engineering from the Georgia Institute of Technology in 1977, a BS in Medical Science from the Emory University School of Medicine Physician Assistant program in 1979, and an MMSc in Career Physician Assistant from Emory in 2006. From 1984 until 2004 he was the program coordinator and a physician assistant at the Georgia Comprehensive Sickle Cell Center at Grady Health System. The center is one of the largest in the world, currently providing primary and emergency care for 1,700 sickle cell patients. He is the web designer of the Sickle Cell Information Center at *www.scinfo.org*. The center won American Academy of Physician Assistants (AAPA) Innovations in Health Care honors in 2000. In 2002, Platt received the Paragon Teacher of the Year Award from the AAPA; in May 2007, the Student Academy of AAPA President's Award; and in 2015 Sickle Cell 101's Sickle Cell Advocate of the Year Award. He is also the co-author of *Overcoming Pain* (Hilton Publishing) and author of *Evidence-Based Medicine for PDAs: A Guide for Practice* (Bartlett and Jones). He is currently assistant professor of medicine and director of admissions at the Emory University School of Medicine Physician Assistant Program.

James Eckman, MD, is a Professor Emeritus of Hematology and Medical Oncology at the Winship Cancer Institute at Emory University School of Medicine. He received his medical training and was appointed to the faculty of University of Minnesota Medical School before being recruited to Emory in 1978. He was committed to establishing a sickle cell program at Grady Memorial Hospital and, after intensive state lobbying for funding in 1984, became Medical Director of the world's first 24-hour comprehensive acute care sickle cell center. The Georgia Comprehensive Sickle Cell Center is currently providing comprehensive health care, anticipatory guidance, and extensive psychosocial support to more than 1,100 active and 3,800 registered adult patients followed for significant sickle cell syndromes. He is an international leader in the care of sickle cell patients and has championed newborn screening for sickle cell disease nationally. This screening has saved the lives of many children with sickle cell disease who would have died from pneumococcal sepsis if timely preventive care with oral penicillin prophylaxis were not started. It was through his efforts that Georgia instituted universal mandatory sickle cell screening for newborns in October of 1998.

Listed as one of America's "Top Doctors" by Castle Connolly Medical Ltd.,

Eckman's dedication to public health delivery of medical services, research, and the study of blood disorders has garnered him widespread recognition, honors, and memberships on numerous national committees. He was recipient of the 2000 and 2002 National Association of Public Hospitals and Health Systems Safety Net Clinician Award, was a 1998 and 2003 finalist for the Atlanta Business Chronicle Healthcare Hero, and was honored in 2006 with a resolution from the Georgia General Assembly for his work.

Lewis L. Hsu, MD, PhD, is a pediatric hematologist dedicated to finding more cures for sickle cell disease and improving treatment and education until more cures can be found. Through his 21 years of leadership of some of the largest sickle cell programs in the country, his immersion in "team science" includes a strong commitment to research because of his bedside appreciation of clinical needs of sickle cell patients. He has published over 70 peer-reviewed papers, contributed to sickle cell websites, games, and smartphone apps that help patients with pain management.

Hsu earned a combined MD-PhD at the University of Rochester School of Medicine and Dentistry. His work on his PhD in biophysics on oxygen transport in microcirculatory networks introduced him to sickle cell disease. After pediatric residency at Yale-New Haven Hospital and fellowship in pediatric hematology-oncology at Children's Hospital of Philadelphia, he joined Eckman and Platt at Emory University in 1994. Hsu was a lead participant in two landmark clinical trials: cures with bone marrow transplantation and stroke prevention in pediatric sickle cell disease ("the STOP study").

Hsu then worked with the National Institutes of Health group of Drs. Mark Gladwin, Greg Kato, and Alan Schechter. With sickle cell mice, Hsu contributed to a growing body of evidence that low availability of nitric oxide is a major feature of the complications of sickle cell disease. He then served in leadership roles in the sickle cell centers at St. Christopher's Hospital for Children in Philadelphia and Children's National Medical Center in Washington, DC, At the University of Illinois at Chicago since 2012, his recent initiatives focus on training community health workers to improve patient care coordination, especially for adolescents and young adults, and with a global perspective on sickle cell. Working closely with adult hematology and emergency medicine and population health, he is building a comprehensive program for pediatric-adult sickle cell care across the lifespan.

CONTRIBUTORS TO EARLIER EDITIONS

Dr. Benjamin Barrah, private practice, Brooklyn, New York.

Melissa Creary, research associate and sickle cell patient, Atlanta, Georgia.

Heidy Dodard, college student and sickle cell patient, Atlanta, Georgia.

Berrutha Harper, president, sickle cell parent patient group.

Dr. Gregorio Hidalgo, attending physician in hematology-oncology at Woodhull Medical and Mental Health Center, Brooklyn, New York.

Mark L'Eplattenier, PA, clinical coordinator and adjunct at SUNY Health Science Center at the Brooklyn Physician Assistant Program.

Sharon Lewis, pre-med student at Brandeis University.

Dr. Beatrice Eleje Onyeador, resident in internal medicine at Woodhull Medical and Mental Health Center, Brooklyn, New York.

Dr. Ehi Philip Osehobo, internist in East Point and Fayetteville, Georgia.

Susan S. Platt, MD, internist, Atlanta, Georgia.

Michelle Rodriguez, patient, Brooklyn, New York.

Allan Sacerdote, MD, chief of adult endocrinology, Woodhull Medical and Mental Health Center, and clinical associate professor of medicine, SUNY Health Science Center, Brooklyn.

Nancy Sacerdote, BA, Brooklyn College; MA, Boston University.

Ingrid Whittaker-Ware, Esq., patient representative and lawyer.

Betty Pace, MD, professor of molecular and cell biology at the University of Texas at Dallas, and author of *Renaissance of Sickle Cell Disease Research in the Genome Era*.

Contributors from The Georgia Comprehensive Sickle Cell Center at Grady Health Center, Atlanta, Georgia

JoAnn Beasley, RN, clinical manager, newborn screening coordinator.

Marietta Collins, PhD, pediatric psychologist.

Beatrice Gee, MD, attending physician; assistant professor of pediatric hematology/oncology, Morehouse School of Medicine

Ann E. Haight, MD, assistant professor of pediatrics, Blood and Marrow Transplant Program, Emory University School of Medicine, Aflac Cancer Center and Blood Disorders Service, Children's Healthcare of Atlanta

Melanie Jacob, MD, MPH, attending physician; assistant professor of hematology/oncology, Winship Cancer Institute, Emory University School of Medicine

Barbara Little, MSN, CNS, psychiatric nurse specialist

Patricia Myler, multimedia teacher and director

Yih-Ming Yang, MD, co-director of pediatric program; professor of pediatrics, associate director and head of education core, Sickle Cell Program, Division of Pediatric Hematology-Oncology, Emory University School of Medicine, Aflac Cancer Center and Blood Disorders Service, Children's Healthcare of Atlanta

CONTENTS

Introduction xi

Part 1: The ABCs of Sickle Cell Disease
1. Understanding the Blood 2
2. Sickle Cell Disease 7
3. Raising Children Who Have Sickle Cell Disease 34

Part 2: Developmental Issues
4. Birth to Six Years 40
5. Six to Twelve Years 54
6. The Teen Years: Thirteen to Eighteen 67
7. Young Adulthood: Nineteen to Thirty-Five 77
8. Adulthood: Thirty-Six to Sixty-Five 90
9. Adults Over Over Sixty-Five 100

Part 3: Living With Sickle Cell Disease
10. General Medical Care 104
11. Pain Assessment and Pain Management 130
12. Managing Depression and Anxiety 145
13. Hydroxyurea and Glutamine Therapy 152
14. Bone Marrow Transplant as a Cure 158
15. Gene Therapy for Sickle Cell Disease *by Betty Pace, MD* 167
16. Participating in Sickle Cell Research 175
17. The Power of One: What You Can Do 181

Part 4: Sickle Cell Trait and Genetics
18. Sickle Cell Trait 190
19. Understanding Genetics 197
20. Genetic Counseling 202

Resources 210
Glossary 234

Bibliography 238
Index 261

INTRODUCTION

...because the life of every creature is its blood.
—Leviticus 17:14

Sickle cell disease is an inherited, lifelong problem that is located within the red blood cells of your body. Red blood cells contain a protein, hemoglobin, that carries oxygen from the lungs to the rest of the body. A single change in the building blocks for hemoglobin causes the red cell to take on a hard sickle shape instead of the normal soft, doughnut shape when it releases oxygen. The sickle shape plugs small blood vessels and blocks blood. It also causes the red blood cell to break apart *(hemolysis)*, and this causes *anemia*, or a low red blood cell count. The body pains and many other complications in people with sickle cell disease are all caused by these blockages and by the anemia.

In the United States, more than 100,000 people have sickle cell disease. It is one of the most common genetic diseases in this country. It is also a serious global problem. Each year, about 1,000 babies are born in America with sickle cell disease.

Today, however, there is much good news. Now people with sickle cell disease live longer and more productive lives, thanks to early detection, preventive medications, better education about the disease, and new treatments.

Many new advances have occurred in the last 25 years to prolong life and even to cure the disease:

- People with sickle cell disease now appear to have an increased life expectancy due especially to new methods for preventing infections, strokes, and organ damage. Many individuals with sickle cell disease are now living to old age.
- Early detection of sickle cell through newborn screening, as well as preventive treatment, education, and therapy, greatly improves the chances of survival from infections and spleen problems from birth to age six. Because of this and other improvements, over 95% of children with sickle cell disease detected by newborn screening and followed in sickle centers are living to become adults.
- The first effective preventive medication (hydroxyurea) has been approved by the Food and Drug Administration. This medication has reduced by half the number of pain episodes experienced, the

- need for hospitalization, and the need for transfusion. Studies now show that it prolongs life.
- In 2017, the US Food and Drug Administration approved Endari (L-glutamine oral powder), developed by Emmaus Life Sciences for use as a preventative in sickle cell patients five years of age and older. This can be given to those taking hydroxyurea.
- Also in 2017, the FDA approved a dissolvable tablet form of hydroxyurea. This helps make it easier to follow the 2014 guideline to offer hydroxyurea to children as young as nine months.
- Bone marrow stem cell transplants now can cure some sickle cell children and adults who have a brother or sister to serve as a matched donor—though only the most serious cases merit the risk of going through this procedure.
- Screening children to find those at high risk of stroke allows effective preventive treatment to stop a stroke from happening.
- There are new ways of fixing the genetic code to correct sickle hemoglobin and new methods of giving the corrected stem cells back to the patient opening the way to a cure for all patients. In March 2017, *The New England Journal of Medicine* published "Gene Therapy in a Patient with Sickle Cell Disease," a report of the first successful case of using gene therapy in a patient with sickle cell disease. In this case, a fifteen-year-old boy in Paris, France, received gene therapy through stem cell transplant, and two years later he had been cured of all the symptoms of severe sickle cell disease.

Despite all of this good news, more needs to be done to educate patients and healthcare providers about sickle cell diseases. Even though it is one of the most common genetic diseases in the United States, research funding for it at all levels is very low because the number of patients is small and, often, the patient's economic status is low as well.

Still, much can be accomplished by motivated people working together for a common goal. The resources in this book can empower you, the reader, to become an informed, active member of the sickle cell community and to change your life and others' for the better.

Because sickle cell disease is genetic, because it involves blood chemistry, and because it can strike many of the body's organs, it is harder to under-

Introduction

stand than diseases that strike single parts of the body.

This book explains clearly what you need to know about sickle cell disease and trait. It is based on the many questions parents, patients, and friends have asked the staff of the Georgia Comprehensive Sickle Cell Center at Grady Memorial Hospital in Atlanta, Georgia, over a period of more than 35 years.

Individuals who inherit one normal and one sickle hemoglobin gene are carriers (often called sickle trait) for the disease; they have no symptoms and do not have a disease but are at risk for having children with the disease. That is why individuals with roots in Africa and many other parts of the world, who are most likely to carry the gene for the disease, need to be tested for sickle cell trait. It is estimated that 3.5 million Americans carry the sickle cell trait. Two people carrying the trait, neither of whom suffer any symptoms, may bring into the world a child with sickle cell disease who does suffer its serious effects.

Patient Stories

We have included stories written by people with sickle cell disease to describe how the disease affects different age groups. From these stories and the stories posted on the Sickle Cell Information Center website, you will get encouragement, instruction, and hope. You may also want to tell your own story on the website, *www.scinfo.org*. The people who tell these stories—parents and people with the disease who have learned to cope with it day by day—are the true heroes of this book.

How to Use This Book

You may want to use this book to address your questions about sickle cell. With the help of the table of contents and index, you can decide which subjects you want to explore first, and get the answers from the book. You may want to journey from cover to cover. This is a preview of what is inside:

Chapter 1 is about the cells flowing in the blood stream and how they work to maintain life.

Chapter 2 explains the different types of sickle cell disease, the worldwide distribution, some preventive tips, and some sickle cell myths.

Chapter 3 is about parenting a child with sickle cell disease, and the options for parents with sickle cell trait.

Chapters 4 through 9 offer a journey from birth to old age, how sickle cell disease affects the body at different stages of life, and the best prevention steps along the way

Chapter 10 is about interacting with the healthcare system, the professionals you may meet, and ways to ensure the best care for your disease. Common medical tests and procedures you may encounter, such as TCD, and blood transfusions, are described.

Chapter 11 is all about pain management and ways you can treat pain.

Chapter 12 is about managing depression, a common condition in those with a lifelong medical problem.

Chapter 13 is about the only approved preventive medication for sickle cell disease and how it can help prevent pain events and complications.

Chapter 14 reviews the first cure offered for sickle cell disease and why it has both good and bad issues to consider.

Chapter 15 is all about gene therapy; now in the research stages, it may have the potential to cure more individuals with sickle cell disease.

Chapter 16 talks about the ongoing current research to find better treatments and what you can do to get involved.

Chapter 17 is the story of how you can make a difference to help those struggling with sickle cell disease.

Chapter 18 is a review of the issues surrounding sickle cell trait.

Chapter 19 is all about genetics: how it determines your eye color and your looks, and how the hemoglobin and your red blood cells are made.

Chapter 20 is about genetic counseling: how your genes could cause medical problems.

The appendices are loaded with resources, from books to websites, to help you learn more. These are exciting times for sickle cell research, new treatments, and hopefully a cure for all with this disease. Keep your hope alive, and follow your destiny.

Allan F. Platt, PA-C, MMSc; James Eckman, MD; and Lewis L. Hsu, MD, PhD
November 2018

PART 1
•
THE ABCs OF SICKLE CELL DISEASE

1

Understanding the Blood

More than five quarts of blood constantly move through the pipes (blood vessels) called arteries that carry blood away from the lungs, and through the veins that carry it back to the lungs. Blood carries food, oxygen, and messages to your body's organs and removes wastes, carbon dioxide, and old cell parts for recycling. Bloods also helps the body heat and cool itself. It is truly the river of life.

PLASMA

Blood is made up of three types of cells, and a liquid called plasma. Plasma contains the water, sugar, salt, hormones, proteins, and minerals necessary to keep cells alive. It is the fluid that carries the cells around the body to where they are needed. Plasma is filtered by the kidney, where urine is made; the liver, where protein is made and stored; and the spleen, where germs and old cells are removed from the blood.

BLOOD CELLS

There are three types of blood cells that circulate in blood vessels: red cells, white cells, and platelets.

Red Cells

Red blood cells are the soft doughnut-shaped (the raised, fluffy kind) cells. They are the "taxi cabs" that carry the oxygen from your lungs to all your living cells. They pick up the waste gas carbon dioxide and carry it back to the lungs for you to breathe out. There are 25 trillion red blood cells in the body at any given instant. They are too small to be seen without the help of a microscope, but they give blood its red color. (For example, there would be about 50 red blood cells in the space of the period at the end of this

Understanding the Blood

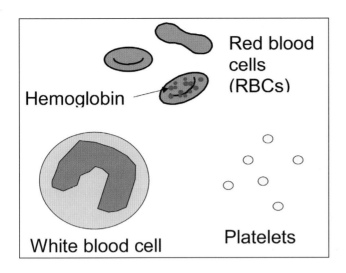

The three types of blood cells

sentence.) The red cell's shape is perfectly designed to travel the narrow capillaries out in the far parts of the body (a capillary is a tiny blood vessel that connects larger blood vessels).

Red cells normally live for 120 days. Then they are destroyed in the spleen and other organs, and the chemicals that make up the cells are recycled.

The red cell is the main actor in the drama of sickle cell disease. One small change in the protein hemoglobin inside the red cell can change its shape and cause all of the problems we will talk about.

White Cells

White blood cells are the defenders of the body. They help capture and fight invading germs and protect the body against foreign cancer cells, viruses, and chemicals. There are different types of white blood cells, each with a different mission and defense location. One type of white cell makes immune protein that fights bacteria, viruses, and foreign proteins that enter the body. Other white blood cells actually eat the germs and kill bad cells. A rising white blood cell count may be the first sign of an infection attacking the body.

The white blood cells in people with sickle cell disease do not attack germs as well as they do in people without sickle cell. The result can be increased infections.

Platelets

Platelets are small cells that plug holes in the blood vessels. When the skin and blood vessels are cut or a hole is made, bleeding occurs. The platelets spring into action and cause the blood to form a jelly-like plug, called a *clot*, to block the hole and stop the bleeding. If there are not enough platelets or they do not work right, you may not stop bleeding. If there are too many platelets, the blood may clot inside blood vessels where there is no hole. This can stop blood flow, causing damage to the tissues in the area. Platelets are more active in people with sickle cell disease than in people without it, leading to increased clotting inside blood vessels where there is no hole.

HEMOGLOBIN

The protein inside the red blood cell that does all of the work is called hemoglobin. It holds the oxygen that is picked up in the lungs, releases it out into the distant tissue, and holds the carbon dioxide for a trip back to the lungs for disposal. It is the hemoglobin that makes the red blood cells red, and gives blood its red color. Hemoglobin with oxygen is bright red, and hemoglobin that has given up its oxygen is dark blue-red.

The way hemoglobin is made is determined by the DNA blueprint that every child inherits from each parent. There are normally three types of hemoglobin in each red blood cell: A, A2, and F or Fetal. Fetal hemoglobin is the main type babies have inside the womb. It tightly holds oxygen so the baby inside the womb can get the oxygen it needs from the mother's blood.

Once the baby is born, fetal hemoglobin is replaced by the adult type, hemoglobin A. Hemoglobin is made according to the genetic blueprint. Normal hemoglobin (hemoglobin A) is made up of two types of protein chains: two alpha chains and two beta chains. Trouble starts when one amino acid called *valine* replaces the normal amino acid called *glutamic acid* in the beta chain.

BONE MARROW

The red cells, white cells, and platelets are all made from stem cells in the bone marrow, inside the big bones of the body. The stem cells make the different cells needed for the blood according to the DNA, a blueprint inherited from each parent.

Anything that harms or stops the bone marrow factory can cause the red cell, white cell, and platelet number to fall, causing the person to be weak, have infections, and suffer increased bleeding.

The only cure available now for sickle cell disease is to destroy a person's bone marrow with medications and replace it, or transplant it, with marrow from another person, such as a brother or sister. This replaces the blood cells that have the sickle cell DNA blueprint with blood cells of the donor, which have a normal DNA blueprint. This is called bone marrow or stem cell transplant.

BLOOD VESSELS

Blood is carried through the miles of tubing in the body called blood vessels. The heart pumps the blood through the vessels that carry oxygenated blood from the lungs to the rest of the body. Arteries carry blood from the heart to smaller arterioles and even smaller capillaries, where the oxygen moves from the blood to the body's cells. Arteries have muscles that control blood flow and pressure by contracting to make the size of the vessel smaller or relaxing to make the opening wider. Some capillaries are smaller than the diameter of the red cell, so red cells must stretch to go through and deliver their life-giving oxygen. If the red cell becomes hard, or rigid, for any reason, it can block blood flow through the capillary. Once the blood flows through the capillaries and delivers the oxygen, it enters small veins that are another place where blood flow problems can occur in sickle cell disease. Usually blood flows from the small veins and then the larger veins for its trip back to the lungs (via the heart) for more oxygen. It is in the slow-flowing small veins where scientists suspect most of the sickling of the red cells occurs.

Sickled red cells are also stickier than non-sickled red cells. They stick to each other and can become stuck to the blood vessel walls, slowing blood flow even more.

THE RED CELL CYCLE

Iron, protein, B vitamins, folate—the building blocks for red blood cells and hemoglobin—are absorbed from the food in the intestines. These nutrients are carried to the bone marrow in the middle of your large bones in the arms, legs, back, and hips. Bone marrow is the blood cell factory that makes red cells, white cells, and platelets. Newly made red cells, called *reticulocytes*, are released into the blood stream and mature over two days. The red cells then are pumped around the body from the lungs to the tissues by the heart.

After its normal 120-day life, the red cell becomes easily damaged and breaks apart. The hemoglobin is released, and is broken down into a chemical called *bilirubin*. The iron and protein from the broken red cell are recycled and reused. Not eating the proper foods, or any bleeding, like menstrual bleeding, can cause low iron, which can make you tired. Bleeding can also cause anemia until the body replaces the lost cells.

The kidneys also help keep red cell production going. Inside the kidneys are cells that sense the level of oxygen in the red cells. If the oxygen level is low, these cells in the kidneys secrete a hormone called *erythropoietin* that travels in the blood stream to the bone marrow and stimulates more red blood cell production. It is like a call from a retail store to a factory to order more products because the shelves are empty. If the kidneys become damaged, the erythropoietin level may fall, and the bone marrow may slow down red blood cell production. This process can now be fixed with injections of manufactured erythropoietin. If doctors need to increase red blood cell production for any reason, they can boost it by giving an injection of one of these hormone replacements.

CAUSES OF ANEMIA

Anemia is a lower-than-normal number of red blood cells and a lower hemoglobin level. Some people get anemia by not eating foods rich in iron or by not getting enough vitamins, proteins, and fats to build the red cells in the bone marrow factory. There are many causes of anemia, and it should be evaluated by your doctor. As you know, the bone marrow factory can be attacked by infections, drugs, or chemicals, causing it to slow down production. Red blood cells can break apart before 120 days, weakening the system. This is called *hemolysis*. In sickle cell disease, red blood cells last only 15 to 20 days instead of the normal 120 days. This is the main cause of anemia in individuals with sickle cell disease. People with different types of sickle cell disease have differing severity of their anemia because of the amount of time that their red cells remain in circulation. Some people have red blood cells that break apart after five days in circulation, some after 50 days or more.

Sickle Cell Disease

Sickle cell is a disease caused by a change in the DNA code blueprint that alters the structure of hemoglobin. This is called a *mutation*. There are four chains in each hemoglobin molecule. Adult hemoglobin has two alpha and two beta chains. The change of one building block (called amino acids) in the beta chain alters the function of the hemoglobin molecule, causing all the problems in the disease.

Hemoglobin is important because it delivers oxygen to all the parts of the body. Sickle hemoglobin does not function properly because hemoglobin molecules stick together after they give up their oxygen in the small blood vessels of the body. Red cells containing sickle hemoglobin then become bent out of shape. This causes them to break apart at a young age and block the blood vessels, causing pain and other complications.

There can be many different changes in the amino acid building block structure of the hemoglobin molecule. These abnormal hemoglobins, called *hemoglobinopathies*, may cause serious disease. *Thalassemias* occur when an inherited hemoglobin problem reduces production of normal alpha or beta chains. If you carry one normal hemoglobin gene and one abnormal hemoglobin gene, you are a carrier for the disease, and may not know it because you are healthy. This is sometimes called having the "trait."

THE TYPES OF HEMOGLOBIN THAT CAUSE SICKLE CELL DISEASE

Sickle cell diseases are caused by hemoglobin (Hb) combinations, including:

- Hb SS (called sickle cell anemia);
- Hb SC;
- Hb Sβ^+ (also spelled as "beta-plus") thalassemia;
- Hb Sβ^0 (also spelled as "beta-zero") thalassemia;

- Hb SD-Punjab, also known as Hb SD-Los Angeles;
- Hb SO-Arab;
- Hb SE; and
- Hb S-HPFH (hereditary persistence of fetal hemoglobin).

Individuals with any of these combinations except HBs-HPFH may have sickle complications, but some are more severe than others. Although we still don't understand why, there are many genetic differences within these hemoglobin combinations that can make one person have a milder course and someone else have a more severe disease.

Hemoglobin SS (Sickle Cell Anemia)
Sickle cell anemia, or Hb SS, is caused by inheriting two sickle genes, one from each parent. This is the most common type of sickle cell disease.

Symptoms may include moderate to severe anemia, increased infections, tissue damage, organ damage, and recurrent pain episodes. The anemia is generally well-tolerated by patients, but the accelerated destruction of red blood cells, with increased formation of bilirubin from the released hemoglobin, does lead to a yellow color in the whites of the eyes, called jaundice, and premature gallstones in many. Treatment with folic acid can prevent increased anemia. Blood transfusions may be needed for severe anemia and other complications. The blocked blood flow to the bones may cause pain episodes, bone infarcts (death of cell elements in the bone and marrow), and avascular necrosis (death of tissue not caused by infection) of the hip and shoulder bones. Sickled red blood cells can become stuck in the spleen, causing it to swell and become painful. This process of blood cells getting trapped in the spleen, along with its enlargement, is called *splenic sequestration*. Blood transfusions made be needed, and removal of the spleen is done in older children when splenic sequestration happens over and over.

Children and some adults may have bacterial infections that are more frequent and severe than in individuals without sickle cell disease. Tissue damage may cause pain and scarring. Strokes may occur in children because of blocked blood flow in blood vessels to the brain. Blocked blood vessels in the eye may lead to bleeding into the eye and loss of vision. As patients age, damage to the lungs causes low oxygen in the blood and breathing problems, and damage to the kidneys causes inability to hold on to water and filter toxins from the blood. Pain episodes, one of the most difficult problems for individuals, can be unpredictable and disruptive to normal life.

Hemoglobin SC

Those with Hb SC disease, the second most common type of sickle cell disease, inherit an Hb C gene from one parent and an Hb S gene from the other. In general, those with Hb SC have a sickle problem that is very similar to sickle cell anemia, though the hemolysis is usually less severe, so the hemoglobin level is higher. Early in life, children have fewer complications; however, adults have increased problems, making Hb SC very similar in severity to sickle cell anemia. The reported average life expectancy of those with Hb SC is about 20 years greater than for those with Hb SS. There is a lower incidence of stroke compared to Hb SS. Having an enlarged spleen is much more common in older children and adults, though it doesn't work normally in fighting infections. This makes splenic sequestration, or the swelling of the spleen, with sickled red blood cells more common later in life than it is with sickle cell anemia. There may be more eye problems, so yearly eye examinations are required, and sometimes even preventive laser surgery is performed. Bone damage from loss of blood flow causes avascular necrosis (AVN) of the hip and shoulder bones, and bone infarctions, making chronic pain more of a problem for older patients. Other symptoms are similar to Hb SS.

Hemoglobin S Beta Thalassemia

Beta thalassemias are inherited disorders in the amount of hemoglobin made in red cells, caused by decreased beta globin production. In most people, the molecule's blueprint structure is normal, but the rate of production is reduced because of a problem communicating between the DNA blueprint to manufacturing machinery that makes the hemoglobin protein. Decreased hemoglobin production causes red blood cells to be smaller than normal and to lack hemoglobin. Beta thalassemia can combine with the sickle hemoglobin to cause sickle beta thalassemia, the third most common type of sickle cell disease.

Sickle beta thalassemia comes in two types: β^0 thalassemia, where no normal hemoglobin A is made, and β^+ thalassemia, where a small amount of hemoglobin A is made.

The severity of the problems related to beta thalassemia is unpredictable. Most people with sickle β^+ thalassemia have working spleens and fewer problems with infection, fewer pain episodes, and less organ damage early in life. They often do very well when they get older; however, some develop complications that are as severe as in individuals with sickle cell anemia.

Those with sickle β^0 thalassemia may have very severe disease that is almost identical to sickle cell anemia or (Hb SS). Hemoglobin levels may be higher and red blood cells smaller on average. Spleens stop working almost as early in childhood, and enlargement of the spleen is more common into than in Hb SS adulthood. Pain episodes, organ damage, and prognosis are very similar to sickle cell anemia Hb SS.

When doing genetic counseling and prenatal diagnosis for sickle cell disease, one must always consider that one partner may be a carrier of a beta thalassemia gene. These carriers are easily missed because their hemoglobin levels, common diagnostic tests, and hemoglobin electrophoresis may be normal or near normal.

Hemoglobin SD, SO, SE
A number of much less common mutated hemoglobin interacts with hemoglobin S to cause clinical symptoms. When individual inherit Hb S from one parent and one of these variants from the other parent, they have variable medical problems. D hemoglobin interacts with Hb S, causing milder sickle cell disease with occasional pain episodes.

Individuals inheriting hemoglobins S and O-Arab have more severe clinical symptoms, much like in Hb SS disease. While the HbE gene is very common in many areas of Southeast Asia, India, and China, HbSE sickle cell disease is not common, and cases are usually milder than HbSS.

Hemoglobin S-HPFH (Hereditary Persistence of Fetal Hemoglobin)
Hemoglobin F (fetal hemoglobin) is the main hemoglobin in the baby's red blood cells before birth. Fetal hemoglobin declines over the first six months of life. This decline is usually slower in those with sickle syndromes, and levels are slightly elevated above normal adult levels. Those with sickle cell anemia have levels from 2% to 20%, with some evidence that those with higher levels have less pain, live longer and have fewer other complications. Fetal hemoglobin directly prevents sickling of Hb S. Individuals with HPFH have high fetal hemoglobin in every red cell, and this makes the clinical problems much milder. The overall health of an individual with Hb S-HPFH is very similar to normal. Hydroxyurea prevents complications in individuals with Hb SS, in part, by increasing fetal hemoglobin levels.

SICKLE HEMOGLOBIN PREVALENCE AROUND THE WORLD

The incidence of hemoglobin S carriers, or sickle cell trait, is about 1 in 68 of the world population. In the black population of the United States, the incidence of is approximately 8%, or about 1 in 12 individuals. The incidence of hemoglobin C trait is about 3%, and, of beta thalassemia trait, almost 1.5%. Between 2,500 and 3,000 individuals with sickle cell diseases are born each year in the United States. The estimates of the incidence of sickle cell syndromes in the black population are:

- sickle cell anemia (Hb SS): 1 in every 375 live black births
- sickle cell hemoglobin C disease (Hb SC): 1 in every 833 black births
- sickle cell beta thalassemia (Hb S beta thal): 1 in every 1,667 black births.

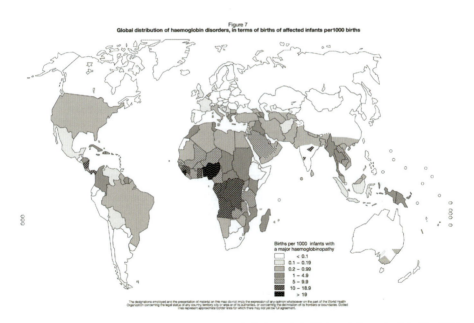

www.who.int/genomics/public/geneticdiseases/en/index2.html#SCA

Incidence of Sickle Cell Disease Worldwide

Brazil 7%–10%	India 9%–38%	Saudi Arabia 5%–25%
Cuba 5%	Jamaica 10%	Southern Italy 10%
Curaçao 12%	Nigeria 24%	Suriname 15%
Ghana 15%	Puerto Rico 5%	Venezuela 11%
Greece 8%–27%	Panama 12%–14%	West Africa 15%–25%

In the Latino population of the United States, the incidence of sickle trait varies widely but averages about 1 in 180 births.

The Distribution

Sickle cell syndromes occur in higher frequency in people from geographic areas where malaria was endemic. This occurs because carriers, like those with sickle cell trait, appear to have some protection against severe malaria infection. The gene for Hb S and thalassemias are common in individuals in parts of Africa, around the Mediterranean Ocean, and in the Middle East and areas of the Western Far East. Genes for Hb E and thalassemias are very common in parts of Asia. In the United States, the disease is more common in African Americans, although it is seen in individuals of almost every ethnic background.

Worldwide View

Sickle cell disease is found in many countries around the world as populations have moved from place to place. Slave trading brought the gene for Hb S to Europe, the United States, South America, Central America, and the Caribbean. Sickle cell has also been found in India and the Arabian Peninsula. Africa still has the highest incidence of trait and disease, with the incidence of sickle cell trait approaching 60% in some areas around the equator.

HOW SICKLE CELL DISEASE SHOWS ITSELF

People with sickle cell disease have hemoglobin that is different in only one way from that of people without sickle cell disease. This simple difference in hemoglobin leads to all of the problems in sickle cell disease.

The difference is the way *sickle hemoglobin* acts when it loses oxygen in the small blood vessels. Sickle hemoglobin without oxygen forms rigid, crystal-like rods called polymers inside the red blood cells that cause cells to take on a sickle shape. Clumping of these sickled red blood cells blocks the blood vessels, slowing blood flow. Loss of blood flow reduces oxygen delivery (ischemia), causes body cells to die (infarction), and causes pain.

Blood cells from individuals with Hb SS are also stickier than those with Hb AA. This adds to blocking of blood flow. Platelets and white blood cells also plug up the blood vessels and further slow blood flow. There is anemia because the red cells don't last as long. There are many other changes that are caused by this sickling and the increased breakdown of the red cells that

Normal red blood cell

Sickled red blood cell

lead to sickle cell pain episodes and most other problems.

Some crises are sudden and severe; others are not. Pain episodes can be caused by low oxygen, infections, dehydration, overheating, cold exposure, your period (menses), and stress.

A newborn with sickle cell disease does not show any signs of sickle cell disease because the fetal hemoglobin is high. As the hemoglobin F decreases during the first six months, the infant may start to have problems. The first symptom of the disorder in infants is often swelling of the hands and feet (hand-foot syndrome, or *acute sickle dactylitis*). This is caused by blocked blood flow, which is caused by sickled red blood cells. This results in a rapid, painful swelling of the bone marrow cavity of the small bones in the hands and feet.

There are three major concerns that arise early in life and justify newborn screening and early preventive care:

- There is an increased risk of have life-threatening infections with certain types of bacterial infections. These can be prevented by vaccination, daily antibiotics, and prompt medical responses to fever.
- Infants and young children are at risk for rapid trapping of the red blood cells in the spleen, called splenic sequestration, that can lead to life-threatening anemia without treatment. Monitoring of the spleen size and hemoglobin level by parents and health professionals has been shown to reduce serious outcomes.
- Young children with sickle cell anemia are at increased risk for strokes, and close monitoring and a yearly simple painless test, transcranial Doppler, can detect those at risk. Strokes can be prevented by regular transfusions of red cells.

There is also evidence that starting hydroxyurea early in life for individuals with sickle cell anemia and sickle β^0 thalassemia can reduce complications like pain episodes and acute chest syndrome and prevent neuropsychological damage.

The Importance of Reading the Signs

Nothing is more important for patients and families than to recognize the symptoms and signs of sickle cell disease complications early and start appropriate actions. Because sickling of the blood may occur anywhere in the body and cause blockages of the blood vessels, sickle cell anemia can affect a wide range of body systems. That is why individuals with sickle cell diseases can develop so many different complications and the disease can vary so much from one person to the next.

Many of the symptoms mimic those of other, more common diseases whose treatment can be quite different. For instance:

- Abdominal pain, in a sickle cell patient, might seem to be the usual pain episode related to the disease; it might, however, be due to splenic sequestration or gallstones—a condition known as *biliary colic*.
- Bone pain in a person with sickle cell disease may be mistaken for a typical pain episode, and the patient or family may first try pain medication at home. On the other hand, that pain could be caused by a serious bone infection known as *osteomyelitis*, which requires different treatment.
- Gallstones occur more frequently in people with sickle cell disease because, as red blood cells are broken down more rapidly, they release hemoglobin, which is converted into bilirubin. This causes the whites of the eyes to be yellow and puts these individuals at risk for gallstones.

In order to deal effectively with sickle cell disease, you should be able to:

- recognize the typical features of a sickle cell an individual with disease;
- recognize the early signs of complications in a previously healthy baby;
- know when to urgently seek medical attention;
- learn to anticipate and understand the differences in appearance and development between children or siblings with sickle cell anemia and others without the disease; and
- learn to allow an individual with disease to grow to their full potential.

PHYSICAL ISSUES

Generally, a child's final height is not affected by sickle cell disease, but the rate of growth during childhood and adolescence is slower. So final height may not be reached until the early twenties. Weight tends to be abnormally low. Bone development is delayed. Sexual maturation takes longer, causing delayed development. Puberty does occur and, as adults, individuals with sickle cell disease have the advantage of not looking as old as others their age. Unfortunately, kids and teens can be cruel, and merciless teasing about delayed growth and sexual development sometimes occurs as a result of ignorance. In severe cases of delayed growth and development, hormonal therapy with estrogen in girls or testosterone in boys may help to reverse the problem of delayed onset of a period in females and delayed maturation of males' sexual organs.

Symptoms of Sickle Cell Disease

Diagnosis	Symptoms	Reason for Symptoms
Anemia	Weakness, tiredness, being more pale, shortness of breath	Reduced survival and/or decreased productions of red cells containing hemoglobin
Infection	Fever, pain in area of infection	Damage to the spleen early in life
Pain episode (crisis)	Sudden severe pain all over or in one spot similar to past episodes	Decreased blood flow in muscle, bones, and other tissues due to sickling
Hand-foot syndrome	Pain, symmetric swelling of hands and feet, crying with movement	Sickling blocks blood flow to hands and feet
Acute chest syndrome	Fever, chest pain, shortness of breath, rapid breathing	Slowing of blood flow to the lungs; infection
Stroke	Headache, weakness on one side, paralysis, difficulty walking, difficulty speaking, dizziness, passing out	Lack of blood flow or bleeding in the brain
Splenic sequestration	Stomach pain, left chest or shoulder pain, spleen larger than usual, weakness, fatigue, paleness	Sickled red cells trapped in the spleen
Gallbladder attacks (cholecystitis)	Increased jaundice (yellow of eyes), pain in stomach, nausea, vomiting, poor appetite, food intolerance	Stones in the gallbladder form because of increase in breakdown of hemoglobin from destroyed red cells
Bone infarction	Localized pain, swelling, and redness over a bone	Prolonged stoppage of blood flow from sickling
Priapism	Spontaneous prolonged painful erection	Blockage of blood flow out of the penis due to sickling
Leg ulcer	Painful skin ulcers on ankle or foot that do not heal	Decreased blood flow in veins, minor skin trauma, sickling, and inflammation.

Diagnosis	Symptoms	Reason for Symptoms
Delay in growth and puberty	Short stature, delayed menses, body hair, voice change	Increased calories needed because of anemia: the need to make red blood cells, and the energy devoted to pump blood faster.
Kidney problems	Having to pass urine frequently, bed wetting, dehydration	Sickle cell damage to kidney cells causes too much water to be passed in urine
Vision problems	Loss of vision, red vision, eye pain, flashes of lights	Bleeding from damaged blood vessels, detached retina
Pulmonary hypertension (High pressure in blood vessels of the heart)	Shortness of breath, fatigue, can't exercise as long	Increased pressure in the lung arteries from heart or lung disease or as a primary problem

PSYCHOSOCIAL ISSUES

Studies have generally shown that individuals with sickle cell disease are well adjusted without significant psychological problems, despite living with this challenging disease. Psychosocial issues, such as depression, low self-esteem, poor family relationships, and social isolation, can arise from being chronically ill. School grades, too, may be lower if students miss many days of class. Chronic pain is a part of these children's lives, but, unfortunately, others sometimes misinterpret such students' reaction to pain as slacking off. Studies also show that some children suffer silent damage to the brain and have learning difficulties. Formal testing for these problems can be very helpful in planning educational activities for these individuals. All children with sickle cell who have significant medical problems should have a special educational plan (Individualized Education Plan or 504 Plan). It is important to have good family support, group support, and medical care to help you with all the issues that you may face.

ECONOMIC ISSUES

The economic impact of sickle cell disease is enormous. Patients can require hospitalization for acute pain crisis, aplastic anemia, stroke, acute chest syndrome, infections, and even priapism. During hospitalization, patients will often need blood transfusions, intravenous fluid therapy, and pain management. The disease also causes additional financial challenges for the parents who often miss work when their child is going to regular appointments, home ill, in the hospital, or getting transfusions and other treatment as an outpatient.

Careful outpatient evaluation, management, and prevention can help curb some of the cost of hospitalization. Antibiotics and immunizations can be given in the first years of life to help minimize infections. Rehabilitative services may also be required. Adults may have problems obtaining and maintaining employment because of frequent absences for illness and healthcare. It is important that vocational choices are realistic given the potential physical limitations and effects of environment that may be present. However, it is also important that every individual is encouraged to plan and pursue their vocational dreams to the maximum extent of their abilities. Individuals with sickle cell disease are teachers, entertainers, lawyers, doctors, politicians, and almost all occupations that do not have very rigorous physical demands.

INFECTIONS

Infections are one of the greatest dangers to those with sickle cell disease early in life. Bacterial infections are the most common cause of death in children during their first five years. Although those under age three are at greatest risk for life-threatening infections, they can be acquired at any age. The spleen is the body's major defense against certain deadly germs. Because the spleen of a person with sickle cell disease doesn't work properly, there is a decreased ability to fight off this type of infection. Serious infections such as blood infections (sepsis), infection surrounding the brain (meningitis), and lung infection (pneumonia) caused by these germs are common. The bones and joints may also become infected.

Infections of the bladder and kidney are more common among people with sickle cell disease. These infections may also be more severe than in those without SCD. Lives can be saved by detecting these infections early and treating them with the proper antibiotic. (See the section on medications within this chapter for more on this topic).

Episodes of pain and other complications can also be caused by common infections found in all children. Viral infections like the common cold, influenza, and stomach flu can cause sickle complications because of fever, inflammation, and dehydration.

PREVENTION OF PROBLEMS: FARMS

The best way to avoid problems is to prevent them from happening. Remember FARMS—the basic principles of prevention in sickle cell disease:

F is for *Fluids and Fever*. Drink plenty of water and manage fever. If you get a fever, see your healthcare provider right away.

A is for *Air*. Make sure you get enough oxygen. Do not smoke or do other things that may damage your lungs. Consult with your doctor before going to high altitudes or flying in unpressurized airplanes.

R is for *Rest*. Get plenty of sleep, do not overdo it, and take plenty of breaks when your body feels tired. Learn to pace yourself.

M is for *prevention Medications*, like daily penicillin for children under six. Consider taking hydroxyurea for pain prevention. The vitamin folic acid is needed to make new red blood. Take all of your medications as directed by your doctor.

S is for *Situations* to avoid, like stress, getting too hot or cold; getting dehydrated; and using tobacco, alcohol, and street drugs. When you exercise and work outdoors, wear the proper clothing for the season. Drink plenty of water, and take frequent rest and water breaks. Carry a water bottle with you, and drink from it often. Avoid swimming pools that are too cold or hot tubs that are too hot.

Do not let peer pressure make you do things you know will make you sick. Avoid emotional stress by pacing projects and work. Avoid situations that you know are upsetting. Join a support group that offers spiritual and emotional support.

Fluids

The simple act of consuming extra water can dramatically delay the sickling effect. Even a little bit of water can make a tremendous difference—drinking 10% more water, for example, can slow down sickling by 1,700%.

It is especially important for children with sickle cell to drink plenty of water because their kidneys cannot hold water in the body very well. Loss of water through urine continues at a high rate all day and all night. It is very easy for people with sickle cell to quickly become dehydrated if they do not drink enough to replace the water lost.

The best fluid is *water*. Other fluids like juice, milk, soup, fruit, or sports drinks are fine, and, to add some variety, so are Popsicles. On the other hand, limit drinks with *caffeine* (cola, coffee), alcohol, or theophylline, (the specific chemical which is found in tea in addition to caffeine). These ingredients make the kidney release even more water into the urine. If your child is fond of cola, tea, or "energy drinks," see if they like the caffeine-free types, or try to limit him or her to no more than two glasses a day.

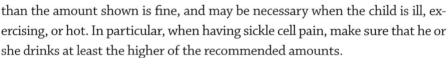

The amount of water you need to drink depends on your size. What pediatricians call the maintenance rate of fluids is the minimum you need to avoid dehydration. Drinking 1.5 times this recommended amount is even better. The chart on the next page indicates how much an individual child should drink. Drinking more than the amount shown is fine, and may be necessary when the child is ill, exercising, or hot. In particular, when having sickle cell pain, make sure that he or she drinks at least the higher of the recommended amounts.

Air

Air means getting enough air—and oxygen—into your lungs and into your red blood cells. The red blood cells with sickle hemoglobin become sickled when the hemoglobin gives up its oxygen. The ways to rob the red cells of oxygen include: smoking, mountain climbing, having asthma or pneumonia, and flying in unpressurized aircraft.

You should not smoke, and, if you do, you should stop. Smoking damages lungs and robs the body of valuable oxygen. Family members who smoke should do so outside and away from the one with sickle cell disease.

Asthma can be treated with medications that open the airways and prevent them from closing. Shortness of breath, fever, cough, or chest pain may all be early signs of pneumonia or acute chest syndrome. One of the medications used to treat asthma, although not as frequently in the past, is theophylline. Because it may cause dehydration, even while improving breathing and oxygenation, its use in sickle cell patients should probably be limited to those situations where other alternatives have been exhausted, and always with good oral or intravenous hydration. If you have any of these symptoms, see your doctor immediately for a complete evaluation.

Commercial airplanes are pressurized and many individuals can fly without difficulty. If you have problems after flying, consider using oxygen on future flights. Do not go to higher altitudes in unpressurized aircraft or hike on high mountains without taking oxygen along. (See the section on air travel.)

Rest

Exercising to exhaustion causes muscles to make *lactic acid*, leading to acidosis. Acidosis increases sickling and may trigger sickle cell pain and other problems. A child with a lower hemoglobin level will reach this state sooner than one with a higher level.

Daily Water Consumption Recommendations

Metric units

Body weight (kilograms)	Recommended range per day (liters)
5	0.5 to 0.7
10	1.0 to 1.4
15	1.2 to 1.8
20	1.4 to 2.2
25	1.5 to 2.3
30	1.7 to 2.5
35	1.8 to 2.7
45	2.0 to 3.0
55	2.3 to 3.4
65	2.5 to 3.8
75	2.8 to 4.1

English units

Body weight (pounds)	Recommended range per day (8-ounce cups)
10	2 to 3
25	4 to 6
30	5 to 8
45	6 to 9
55	7 to 10
75	8 to 11
100	9 to 13
130	10 to 15
150	11 to 17
175	12 to 18

To avoid exhaustion, children with sickle cell should take frequent breaks when playing. During vigorous play, taking a break every 15 to 20 minutes both to rest and to drink usually will allow them to continue their activities without developing lactic acidosis. One young man, for example, often developed sickle cell pain if he played basketball for 30 minutes straight. However, he found that he could cut down on his pain episodes by playing the first quarter of a basketball game, resting the second quarter, playing the third, and resting the fourth. Physical education teachers or coaches may need a note from the family or doctor to explain this situation.

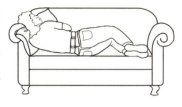

Medical Care and Medications

Sickle cell patients should be under the care of a medical team that understands sickle cell disease. Parents should know how to check for a fever, because this signals the possibility of a serious infection. All newborn babies with sickle cell disease should be placed on daily penicillin (or similar antibiotic) to prevent serious infections. All of the usual childhood immunizations should be given, plus the pneumococcal vaccine. There is growing evidence that taking hydroxyurea daily prevents pain and other complications and may increase life expectancy.

The following are general guidelines to keep the sickle cell patient healthy:

- Take the vitamin folic acid (folate) daily to help make new red cells.
- Take daily penicillin (or equivalent antibiotic) until age six to prevent serious infection.
- Drink plenty of water daily (8–10 glasses for adults).
- Avoid extremes of temperatures.
- Avoid overexertion and stress.
- Get plenty of rest.
- Stay current with your physician-recommended vaccinations from childhood through adulthood.
- Get regular checkups from expert healthcare providers.

Patients and families should watch for the following conditions that need an urgent medical evaluation:

- Fever
- Chest pain

- Shortness of breath
- Increasing tiredness
- Abdominal swelling
- Unusual headache
- Any sudden weakness or loss of feeling
- Pain that will not go away with home treatment
- Priapism (painful erection that will not go down)
- Sudden vision change

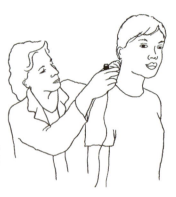

Situations

Many individuals report that stress brings on pain episodes, so you should learn ways of reducing stress. Being either chilled or overheated changes the blood flow patterns in the body and can lead to sickle cell pain. When the weather is cold, dress your child warmly. When the weather is hot and he or she is spending time outside, make sure your child takes frequent breaks in the shade or an air-conditioned room. Many people find that swimming in unheated water can chill the body quickly and trigger sickle cell pain. That's why children with sickle cell should take rest breaks often to dry off and warm up.

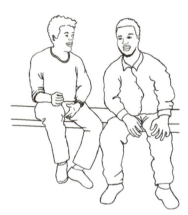

When the weather is changing quickly or your activities will take you from the hot outdoors to cool air-conditioning, make sure to dress your child in layers so that you can help regulate his or her temperature. A sweat suit or warm-up outfit can be very helpful for staying warm before and after exercise.

Avoid using illegal drugs, such as cocaine; these are deadly to those without sickle cell disease and many times more deadly for those with it. Alcohol should also be avoided because it dehydrates the body and makes the blood more acidic—just the right conditions to increase sickling.

IMMUNIZATIONS

Because infections often trigger pain and other sickle cell crises, it is vitally important that you get immunized against certain preventable serious infections. Recommended immunizations include:

- pneumococcal (a common cause of pneumonia);
- annual influenza vaccine;
- hemophilus influenza type B (a common cause of sore throats, sinus and middle ear infections, acute bronchitis, and pneumonia); and
- meningococcus (a common cause of meningitis).

Immunizations should be given only when patients are in the best possible health. Immunizations should not be given when a sniffle, cold, or flu is present because then immunizations will more likely cause an unpleasant, or possibly dangerous, reaction. They may also be less effective.

Immunizations should, if possible, be given when the patient is young, before much damage to the spleen has occurred. Early detection and aggressive treatment of infection is key to preventing and/or reducing the severity of sickle crises. A current listing of all recommended vaccines is available at the Centers for Disease Control and Prevention's website at *www.cdc.gov*.

Pneumococcal Vaccine

Two types of pneumococcal vaccines offer protection against 90% of the strains that cause serious infection in the United States. Conjugated pneumococcal vaccine, Prevnar 13, can be given as early as two months after birth, followed by two more doses six to eight weeks apart and a booster dose at 12 months. This is followed by Pneumovax at ages two and five years. Consult current recommendations at *www.cdc.gov*.

Meningococcal Vaccine

Meningococcal vaccines are a little complicated because there are different vaccines against a broad range of meningococcus strains. The meningococcal conjugate vaccine (MCV-4) is now recommended for infants with sickle cell disease, with booster doses recommended every five years. New vaccines for serogroup B meningococcal (MenB) are available, and vaccination against MenB is recommended for teenagers with sickle cell and for people exposed to someone with meningococcal infection. Patients traveling to areas where meningococcal disease is epidemic (check with your airport's travel clinic or at *www.cdc.gov*) should also receive one dose of the vaccine before leaving.

Household contacts of patients with meningococcal infection are at increased risk of infection themselves and should receive preventive treatment with the antibiotic rifampin. For those who are unable to tolerate rifampin, there are several alternative antibiotics:

- ciprofloxacin;
- profloxacin; and
- ceftriaxone—for pregnant women or children under 12 years old.

Immunization for meningococcal infection is recommended not only for those who live with infected persons but for anyone who has had close contact with an infected patient in settings such as nursery schools, day care centers, and camps, or for anyone who has had oral contact with an infected patient. Oral contact includes actions such as kissing, mouth-to-mouth resuscitation, or sharing of the same utensil, plate, glass, cup, or toothbrush. These recommendations can change, so check *www.cdc.gov* for the current CDC recommendations you should follow.

MALARIA PREVENTION

The prevention of malaria is complex and constantly changing based on the prevalence of malaria and drug resistant malaria. Individuals with sickle cell disease and sickle cell trait have the same risk of being infected as the general population. **You are not protected from malaria infection because you have sickle trait or disease.** Individuals with sickle cell disease commonly become extremely ill and often die from malaria infection. Preventing infection when you travel to areas where malaria is common is extremely important.

The first thing you can do for yourself is to avoid being bitten by mosquitoes, which carry the disease. Measures you can take:

- Avoid travel, if possible, to areas where malaria is common.
- Avoid being outdoors in such areas at peak mosquito feeding times (dusk and dawn).
- Use an effective insect repellent regularly in such areas. DEET is one. Increased dietary garlic and brewer's yeast have also been described as excellent natural additional insect repellents.
- Wear long pants and long sleeves in endemic areas (admittedly tough in the hot tropical and subtropical areas where malaria is common).
- Use window screens.
- Use bed netting treated with the chemical permethrin (recently shown to reduce malaria deaths in Africa).

Taking certain medications to prevent malaria infections is recommended when traveling to areas where malaria is common. Consult the CDC or a clinic that specializes in travel medicine.

For current recommendations and more detailed information about malaria, see the Appendix and the CDC website.

LIFE EXPECTANCY

The most current information available from scientific articles is listed, and is the information we use. But keep in mind that life expectancy for those with sickle cell disease keeps going up with newer treatments, better prevention, more education, genetics, healthy living, and good healthcare. In the Georgia Comprehensive Sickle Cell Center, we see several patients in their 50s, 60s, and 70s. We even have an 80-year-old who drops in for monitoring and treatment.

Median Survival of Individuals of All Ages with Sickle Cell Disease Based on Sickle Cell Disease Type and Sex[1]

Sex	Genotype	Median Survival
Male	Hb SS	42 years
Female	Hb SS	48 years
Male	Hb SC	60 years
Female	Hb SC	68 years

When looking at the survival table, remember that the median is the middle point in the survival range. **IT IS NOT THE AGE AT WHICH YOU ARE LIKELY TO DIE.** It simply means that half of patients lived to be less than that age, and half lived past that age. Also, the older you are, the longer you are expected to live. Individuals with sickle cell disease should be encouraged to live every day to the fullest and prepare for a life into adulthood. Preparation should be made for work, marriage, hobbies, and meaningful contributions to society. Our patient population includes ministers, lawyers, teachers, computer programmers, artists, moms, and dads.

MYTHS EXPLODED

Myth: Sickle cell is like a cold, and you can catch it from someone with the disease.
Truth: You cannot catch sickle cell disease; it is genetic. Only people who are born with this genetic defect can have it. It is lifelong and is present at birth.

---

[1] Platt, OS, et al. "Mortality in sickle cell disease. Life expectancy and risk factors for early death." *New England Journal of Medicine* 330, no. 23 (1994): 1639–1644.

Myth: You must be black to have sickle cell disease.
Truth: Sickle cell is a disease that affects people of all different racial and ethnic backgrounds. The national poster child for sickle cell disease one year was a blonde, blue-eyed Caucasian girl. Many Hispanic people have sickle cell disease. All newborns should be screened at birth for hemoglobin traits and disease.

Myth: If our child has the disease, it means that she got the sickle cell gene from both my spouse and me.
Truth: This is true for sickle cell anemia, Hb SS, but there are other types in which only one parent has passed on the sickle cell gene and the other has passed on a gene for another hemoglobin disorder, such as hemoglobin C, D, E, O, or thalassemia, that interacts with sickle hemoglobin to produce sickle cell disease. This trait may be unknown to the partner.

Myth: Sickle cell trait is not important; it doesn't do anything.
Truth: Sickle cell trait causes you and your child with sickle trait to be at risk for having a child with sickle cell disease if the other parent has sickle trait, thalassemia, or other hemoglobins like C, D, E, or O. In this situation, the risk of a child being born with sickle cell disease is one in four with each pregnancy. If your child and his or her spouse both have sickle cell trait, they should be aware that their children could be born with sickle cell disease. Individuals with sickle cell trait almost never have problems from the trait. Because sickle cell trait is so common, many common disorders occur in individuals who also have sickle trait. The best evidence available suggests that almost all of these disorders are caused by chance and are not truly complications of sickle trait. Although it is uncommon, sickle trait does appear to cause blood to appear in the urine under extremely severe conditions at the limits of human endurance, such as military training or exercise at a high altitude. For example, people with the trait can develop episodes of pain, splenic sequestration, and an increased risk of sudden death when they exercise very hard and become dehydrated in heat or at high altitude. Blood clots may also be more common in those with sickle trait. For more information about sickle trait, read Chapter 18.

Myth: People with sickle cell disease or sickle cell trait cannot get malaria.
Truth: People with sickle cell disease and trait get malaria as easily as those without the disease or trait. Malaria is very severe and often fatal in someone with sickle cell disease. However, people with sickle cell trait tend to survive malaria better than those without the trait, but still can get very sick and die (see malaria prevention).

Myth: People with sickle cell will not live past the teenage years.
Truth: Life expectancy in sickle cell disease has increased thanks to newborn screening and several recent advances in care—in particular, better management of strokes, and new methods for preventing infections and treating fever. The expectation is that greater than 95% of individuals with sickle cell anemia and sickle β^0 thalassemia will live to be adults. The outlook is even better for those with Hb SC and Sβ^+ thalassemia. An effective medication to improve sickle cell—hydroxyurea—was approved by the Food and Drug Administration more than 20 years ago for adults, and in 2017 for children. It clearly reduces pain crisis, acute chest syndrome and anemia in children and adults. Studies have shown it is safe and effective in children with sickle cell disease. New data suggests it also may increase life-expectancy. A recent consensus conference by the National Institutes of Health concluded that hydroxyurea is used by too few people with sickle cell disease who should be on the drug, and 2014 NHLBI guidelines suggest offering hydroxyurea to children as young as nine months.

Myth: There is no cure for sickle cell disease.
Truth: As of 2018, more than 1,600 sickle cell patients have been cured by bone marrow stem cell transplant. For more information about this procedure, see Chapter 14.

Myth: Sickle cell patients and their families cannot chart their own destiny.
Truth: Patients and families need to strike a balance between completely denying the presence of the disease and living in a bubble. Learning about preventive measures and applying them can prevent complications and pain.

Myth: My child has hemoglobin SC; this is the same as sickle cell trait.
Truth: Hemoglobin SC is very definitely a type of sickle cell disease, and it does have symptoms. Painful episodes for a population of children with Hb SC may not be as severe or frequent as in Hb SS, but there is wide variation between individuals. After childhood, the complications of Hb SC patients increase so that the disease becomes very similar in severity to adults with Hb SS. Sickle cell

pain typically involves bones, including joints and the skull, but it can affect nearly any part of the body. In older school-age children and adolescents with Hb SC, there is a high rate of two complications of sickle cell disease: damage to the joints (due to sickled cells interfering with blood flow to the heads of the femur and humerus), and damage to the blood vessels of the retina (lining of the eye) that can cause bleeding. We routinely check Hb SC children for these problems and recommend annual retinal examination by an ophthalmologist after age eight. Other sickle cell complications such as stroke, acute lung problems, and aplastic crisis are less frequent in Hb SC than Hb SS, but they can still occur.

CLIMATE

There are some reports that the mild climate of the tropics may benefit sickle cell patients. It is known that exposure to extreme cold or hot temperatures can promote sickling. Proper clothing and protection from the temperature is necessary in climates that have temperature extremes. In dry climates, drinking a lot of water is important to keep up with water losses.

SPORTS

Moderate exercise is generally a good idea, but watch out for dehydration and exhaustion.

We encourage activities that require concentration and skill rather than endurance. Golf, martial arts, skateboarding, bowling, table tennis, and fencing might be good choices.

Swimming in a heated pool may also be tolerated, but chilling on exit and any cold pool may cause pain crisis and other problems. Exercise in a heated pool may be beneficial because of the low impact on knees and hip joints. "Extreme" or endurance sports (long-distance competitive racing, for example), which push the body to exhaustion and cause dehydration, are likely to cause problems. Sports that involve cold temperatures (skiing, sky diving) or low oxygen (mountain climbing) will probably trigger sickle cell pain. It is important to be physically active but very smart to avoid vigorous exercise to exhaustion or any activity that consistently results in pain or other symptoms.

Common triggers for increased sickle cell pain are dehydration, temperature extremes (both cold and heat), low oxygen, exhaustion (lactic acidosis), infection, and stress. Sickle cell pains show up in certain places in the body because of vaso-occlusion, or blood-flow blockage. Generally, pain affects the long bones, such as those in the arms and legs, and the vertebrae.

Active youngsters need to pay particular attention to the hip, where avascular necrosis is extremely common in young adults with sickle cell. This can be accelerated by repetitive injury from high-impact sports. Pain in the hip or knee should be evaluated by an orthopedist with sickle cell experience. Patients with diagnosed avascular necrosis of the hip should not participate in sports that involve repetitive jumping (basketball, dance, and gymnastics, to name a few) that may cause further injury to the hip joint.

Hydration before, during, and after sports activity is critical. Rest breaks every 20 minutes to avoid acidosis and for hydration should be scheduled. For sprains and strains, avoid using ice. Try instead applying a cool, not cold, compress to reduce swelling without causing the risk of vasoconstriction, which can aggravate pain in the area. If the patient has a much-enlarged spleen, contact sports (football, hockey, lacrosse, etc.) present a risk of rupturing the organ, but the level of danger depends on the amount of trauma to the left upper belly.

AIR TRAVEL AND ALTITUDE EXPOSURE

In some patients, sickle pain episodes are caused by flying. The major problem we have seen is pain crisis shortly after the flight. Some of our patients have traveled all over the world without problems.

The major problem is a decrease in oxygen in the cabin air. The aircraft may be only pressurized to between 6,000 and 8,000 feet. At 8,000 feet, there is 25% less oxygen than at sea level, which is low enough to get some people with sickle cell in trouble. The other problem related to air travel is dehydration. The humidity in the aircraft can be very low, and fluid intake needs to be markedly increased before and during the flight.

If you have had trouble flying, we would recommend supplemental oxygen at 2 liters/minute or 120 liters/hour. Most airlines now require passengers to provide their own Federal Aviation Administration-approved oxygen equipment, and this needs to be arranged well in advance of planned travel. Oxygen concentrator machines are easier to manage than oxygen tanks.

Ask the airline for an aisle seat so that you can stretch your muscles and get to the bathroom easily. Plan to drink a pint of water an hour during the flight. You may need to carry on the water you will need because airlines generally do not provide the amount of fluid needed. Carry empty water bottles through security and fill them near the gates. Many airports now have fill stations for water in the gate areas.

When traveling, make sure you have a supply of all of the medicines you will need during your trip. You also should have a letter from your doctor that summarizes your disease complications, your most recent laboratory results, your current medications, and a detailed treatment plan for pain episodes so that, if illness occurs, the treating doctors will know average values. Be sure all vaccinations are up to date and you have recommended vaccinations for foreign travel.

Traveling to areas above 7,000 feet in elevation may cause sickle complications. Check with your doctor before going.

HEALTHY DIET, "NATURAL TREATMENT"

While everyone needs to think about what they eat, a healthy diet is even more important for children with sickle cell disease. These key principles are good to follow:

- Children with sickle cell have the same basic nutritional requirements as anyone else.
- The Choose MyPlate program developed by the federal government is a useful guide (*www.choosemyplate.gov*).
- A healthy diet helps every child grow well and avoid illness.
- Learning and practicing good eating habits while still young can help prevent many diseases later in life, such as diabetes, hypertension, heart disease, stroke, and cancer.
- So far, researchers believe that the same antioxidants and anti-clotting foods that help prevent heart disease, stroke, and cancer also help reduce health problems caused by sickle cell disease.
- A diet rich in fruits and fresh vegetables is very important to provide folic acid. Daily folic acid may be recommended if you do not include healthy portions of these in every meal.
- Extra fluids are very important. Avoiding dehydration is a good way to decrease the likelihood of pain crises.

Recent research shows that children with sickle cell SS and Sβ^0 thalassemia need approximately 20% more calories than other children because of the extra energy needed to make new red blood cells. The calories contained in our food are converted by our bodies into energy that is used to help us do our daily activities, grow, and ward off infection. Not getting enough calories may lead to delays in growth and maturation.

Be sure your child snacks on healthy foods, such as fruits, vegetables, and grains, not just junk food. Work in some additional calories (and protein) by putting peanut butter on celery or carrots; adding cheese, nuts, or wheat germ to appropriate foods; making milkshakes or yogurt smoothies; and serving pudding or instant breakfast drinks. Many African-American and other minority youngsters and adults are lactose intolerant, meaning they lack an intestinal enzyme called lactase, which breaks down lactose, the natural sugar in milk and dairy products. Lactose intolerance causes gas pains, cramps, and diarrhea after consuming milk or dairy products. Yogurt is the dairy product least likely to cause problems because it contains a friendly bacterium called *Lactobacillus*, which removes most of the lactose from the yogurt. You can also purchase Lactaid brand milk, which has the enzyme added, or take Lactaid drops about 30 minutes before eating dairy products. The drops may also be added to normal milk to change it into Lactaid milk, but allow at least 30 minutes for the drops to work.

Even though children with sickle cell need more calories, it is just as important for them to maintain a normal weight. Being overweight increases the stress on bones and joints, causing more chronic pain in older individuals.

Constipation may be an unfortunate side effect of some of the medications required for the treatment of sickle cell pain. Drinking lots of fluids and consuming plenty of fiber, such as that found in whole grains, fruits, and vegetables, will help prevent or treat constipation. When opiate pain medicines are used, you may need a stool softener as well as a high-fiber diet. You must also drink plenty of water for these to be effective.

People with sickle cell disease need extra folic acid (also known as *folate* or *vitamin B*) to produce red blood cells more quickly. This can be found in foods such as green leafy vegetables, grains, and fresh fruits. You also should consult your child's doctor about whether or not to give a folic acid supplement and, if so, how much your child should take.

Doctors are also studying some other nutrients and foods that might aid people with sickle cell. These include omega fatty acids, magnesium, zinc, African yams, antioxidants, and certain herbs. Eating foods rich in L-arginine like miso, yogurt, and soy protein may increase production of nitric oxide, which keeps blood vessels relaxed, increasing blood flow. Ask your doctor to keep you posted on research updates as they become available.

TEACHER/EMPLOYER GUIDE

Individuals with sickle cell disease may miss more days at school or work because of severe pain episodes caused by the blockage of blood flow to body organs or bones. Such episodes may require treatment at home or in a hospital setting. Below is a guide that can be typed in a letter for your teachers and/or employers. (This guide is on the Sickle Cell Information Center website, *www.scinfo.org*, and can be printed directly from the site.)

- Makeup work for students should be provided to keep the student current with assignments. A hospital- or home-based teacher may be required if the student has prolonged complications.
- Pain episodes may be prevented by allowing the individual to keep well hydrated with water. Do not limit the person's access to water, as his or her requirements are increased. They will likely need frequent bathroom breaks because of mild damage to their kidneys.
- Pain episodes may also be prevented by not allowing the individual to become overheated or exposed to cold temperatures.
- Because of their anemia, individuals with sickle cell may tire before others, and a rest period may be appropriate. Encourage gym and sports participation, but let the person stop and drink fluids without undue attention.
- Sickle cell disease is a lifelong illness that may impair academic performance. Problems should be identified and addressed with appropriate testing as they would be for any child. This is especially important in individuals with sickle cell because they need to be prepared to be successful in vocations that do not require heavy physical labor. Most students with sickle cell disease need an Individual Education Plan (IEP) and many will benefit from a 504 Plan. Parents and teachers should be proactive in assuring students with sickle cell disease have the educational resources they need to reach their full potential.

- Individuals with sickle cell disease may have a yellow tint to their eyes because of increased breakdown of their red blood cells. They also may have a shorter stature and delayed puberty from anemia. Teachers need to be sensitive to the teasing and other bullying that may result.

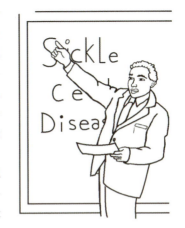

- Those with sickle cell should be treated as normally as possible, with awareness that they may have intermittent episodes of pain, infection, or fatigue. These can be treated and sometimes prevented through adequate water intake and avoiding temperature extremes and overexertion.
- Learn about sickle cell, and understand the challenges that may be faced. Have a plan of action with the individual and their parents to do to keep them productive and complication free.

WHAT YOU CAN DO

- Learn about sickle cell disease from a local sickle cell community-based organization and the student's healthcare provider.
- Invite a speaker from your local sickle cell foundation or clinic to educate the entire class or staff about sickle cell.
- Become involved in public awareness events like walks, fun runs, kids' camp, and fundraisers.
- Encourage blood donations and blood drives in your community. Many with sickle cell need transfusions to prevent childhood strokes and other complications.
- Encourage people to register as potential donors in bone marrow registries. People with sickle cell can benefit from transplants.
- Support sickle cell research to provide new treatments.
- Encourage sickle cell patients to be the best they can be.

3

Raising Children Who Have Sickle Cell Disease

Train a child in the way he should go,
and when he is old he will not turn from it.
—Proverbs 22:6

Parents whose children have sickle cell disease face special problems and pressures. In this chapter, we'll talk about some of these. We'll also tell you how to work with your healthcare provider. Finally, we will make some suggestions about how to talk to your child.

WHAT IS REQUIRED OF THE PARENT

Parenting is the most rewarding job, but it is also one of the toughest. Bringing up an African-American or other minority youngster can be tougher still. While the opportunities are great for a minority child born today, the child also faces great dangers from racism in the larger society and from the poverty, drugs, and violence that devastate many minority communities. The disease may cause your child to miss school, visit the doctor frequently, need hospitalizations, take medications, and require special treatments like transfusion.

No wonder, then, that the parent of a child with a serious, long-term illness like sickle cell disease is often overburdened. Look at what this disease requires of such a parent:

- First, you must become a student of the disease. That means you must get to know the preventive techniques available and how to get medical help when it is needed. It also means learning to recognize and treat potential problems before they get serious.

- ◆ Second, you must accept the increased financial and time commitment required to deal with the disease in your child.
- ◆ Third, you must encourage your child's growth and independence without becoming overprotective.
- ◆ Fourth, you must become an advocate for your child at school, work, and the community.
- ◆ Finally, if you have more than one child, you must stretch yourself to give enough attention to your healthy children. Otherwise, they are likely to become jealous of the child with sickle cell disease.

In short, sickle cell disease calls on all the parents' wisdom and love.

Sometimes, it may seem to call on more than any one human being could possibly have. Parents may feel that their own hold on ordinary life is slipping away. Careers can be compromised because, just as your child is likely to experience long and frequent absences from school, you, as parent, may experience long and frequent absences from work to care for your child when he or she becomes ill. This uncertainty may affect your choice of career, your ability to do your job well, your chance to be promoted, or even where it is wise to live. Even if your company allows family leave, such policies often don't make up for lost job income.

Though family and friends often form a support community around those who suffer, parents facing their human burdens, day after day, may sometimes feel alone. It is very important that family, friends, and colleagues know you have a child with sickle cell disease and what that means for you.

The fact is you are not alone. There are many public and private resources that can help you.

PARENTAL GUILT

Parents of a child with sickle cell disease feel guilty because they have passed on "bad" genes to their child. This is common but not helpful in coping with your situation or raising your child. The fact that your child has sickle cell disease is beyond your control. It is important to get through this, and talking to close friends, family others with children who have sickle cell disease, clergy, and psychologists helps you resolve these feelings and understand it not your fault. It is vital to take care of your own health so you can devote your efforts to raising your special child. It is also important to understand that your spouse may have similar feelings, and your other children may feel guilty because they do not have sickle cell disease.

SUPPORT NETWORKING

As long as children with sickle cell disease do come into the world, they deserve to get the best, most loving care. By drawing on the education, support, and networking other people can provide, parents can anticipate problems and deal with them before they get too big.

One of a parent's first obligations is to know what to expect at each stage of a child's illness and to recognize problems at their earliest stages, when they can be dealt with most effectively. Managing a disease means knowing the best ways to avoid serious symptoms or still more serious complications. Knowing what to expect and not being caught off guard means the parent can react earlier, in a calmer frame of mind, and prevent some emergencies.

It is also important to understand that there are things that can be done to prevent having another child with sickle cell disease. Because parents have a child with sickle cell disease, both carry a gene for sickle cell diseases and are at risk for having more children with sickle cell disease. In fact, the risk is 25%, or 1 in 4 with each pregnancy. It is very important to be tested to see what type of hemoglobin disorders you and your partner have. It is also important to get genetic counseling to know your risks and options for future pregnancies.

TALKING TO YOUR CHILD

The most common problem your child may have is pain. When your child is old enough to understand, talk to him or her about telling you when it hurts. Love, hugs, and reassurance are great ways to ease the pain and go a long way to quiet fears. There will be a day when your child will want to know why he or she is different from other children. That is the time to begin the lifelong journey of teaching your child about sickle cell. Denying, minimizing, ignoring, and running away from the facts will only hurt your child in the long run. Learn all you can so you can fill your child with life-saving knowledge. Tell your child about the blood cells. Show pictures and drawings the child can relate to. Tell your child why it's so important to drink a lot of water, keep warm in cold weather and cool in hot weather, and how not to become over-tired. Encourage your child with play, games that challenge the mind, and reading. Limit television time, and encourage reading. Talk about careers that challenge the mind and don't strain the body.

Teaching your child openly and honestly to talk to you about pain is essential. If that communication is managed well, your child won't complain of pain in order to avoid school, homework, or chores.

Let your child know that he or she will have lots of help in being his or her best, and will have a full life ahead. There will be some stormy days, to be sure, but if the atmosphere is honest and informed, there will be far more sunny ones. Always set your expectations high for your child and teach him or her to always strive for the best, even when not feeling very good. Almost all well adjusted, successful sickle cell patients relate that their parents raised them with the same expectations and discipline as they did for their healthy siblings.

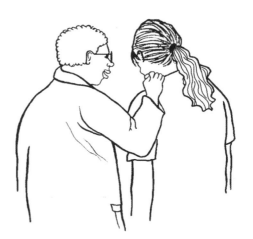

Partner with your child's healthcare providers to learn what to discuss with your child. These specialists may offer tips, books, pictures, videos, and other materials that will make teaching fun and understandable.

Be an example for your child. What you do and how you act has a greater impact than what you say. Children follow your footsteps. If they see you calling in sick to work when you have other plans, they will repeat the pattern and use the disease as an excuse to avoid school or other responsibilities. *Be an example of responsibility, caring, giving, and hope.* This will speak volumes to your child, and you will see the seeds you have planted come to bloom in your child's life.

Take time to have family fun with outings, trips, and activities. It is critical to have the child with sickle cell disease fit into the family unit and not have the other siblings become resentful or neglected.

FINANCING YOUR CHILD'S CARE

Medical costs can be huge for a child with sickle cell disease. Most of the treatment programs we've talked about include social workers who will help you plan the best way to finance your child's care.

Programs like Medicaid and SCHIP are currently available in all states and territories of the United States, as well as Washington, DC. These can pay for practically all of your child's medical care if you qualify. The specific requirements an individual or family must meet to qualify vary from state to state. The best source of information on your state's requirements is a social worker or the local Medicaid office.

Medicaid's stated policy now is to try to eventually enroll most subscribers into Medicaid-HMOs, but patients or their parents can apply for exemptions, which are usually granted in the case of serious, chronic illnesses, like sickle cell disease.

Upon the passage of the Affordable Care Act in 2010, individuals with sickle cell disease and their families got better access to healthcare coverage. As the law stands currently, an insurance company cannot deny healthcare coverage or charge higher rates if a patient has a pre-existing condition like sickle cell disease. In addition, young adults are allowed to stay on their parents' insurance until the age of 26. Many programs to improve management are being established through Centers for Medicare & Medicaid Services' (CMS) Innovation Centers. However, it is important to note that the Affordable Care Act has regularly been challenged by legislators in Congress, so there is the possibility that these protections may one day cease to exist.

For those who earn too much to qualify for Medicaid but who do not have insurance coverage, the options may narrow to community or county hospitals and healthcare centers. These facilities can have excellent care. Seek those hospitals affiliated with medical schools and teaching programs. This is where some of the best treatment is available. The fact is that help is available. If you don't find it at first, keep looking. You will find it eventually.

PART 2

•

DEVELOPMENTAL ISSUES

4

Birth to Six Years

The symptoms of sickle cell disease and its treatment change over the course of the patient's life. In the next chapters, we will talk about these stages of development, beginning with infancy and early childhood.

Let's start with what parents and healthcare providers need to be focused on. First, the clinical issues, period by period.

CLINICAL ISSUES

Birth to 6 Months
- Have the child's hemoglobin electrophoresis done to confirm the sickle cell diagnosis.
- Find a sickle cell clinic, or see a physician with sickle cell experience who will work with your child's primary physician.
- Learn all you can about sickle cell disease symptoms and prevention.
- Schedule physician clinic examinations once a month, usually when immunizations are due.
- Begin giving the child penicillin, 125 mg liquid by mouth twice a day, at least by two months of age.
- Learn how to recognize fever, how to take temperature, respond to fever, and the importance of penicillin.
- Learn all you can about and practice good well-baby care.
- Learn how to palpate the spleen and record its size.
- Get appropriate immunizations when they are due, especially the pneumococcal and meningococcal vaccines.
- It is normal for you to grieve about your child having sickle cell disease. Share that grief by talking to family, friends, clergy, your child's

doctor, community-based sickle cell organizations, or counselors.
- Have your extended family tested for sickle cell, and make a family pedigree.
- Meet with a genetic counselor.

6 Months to 1 Year
- Begin giving the child folic acid (1 mg) every day if it is prescribed.
- Learn about nutrition, prevention of complications and accidents, recognizing illness, measuring spleen size, hand-foot syndrome, and spleen sequestration.
- Schedule clinic visits for every two months.
- Continue having all scheduled immunizations.
- Ask your doctor whether hydroxyurea is suitable for your child.
- Join a support group, or talk to other parents with sickle cell disease infants.
- Report concerns and issues to your physician.

1 to 2 Years
- Continue all immunizations.
- Discuss with your doctor pain control, growth/development, and issues related to lifelong disease.
- Schedule clinic visits every three months.
- Each clinic visit should include a physical examination, complete blood count, and reticulocyte count.
- Get the pneumococcal vaccine, 23-valent, at age two.
- Blood chemistries should be done twice a year.
- Learn and watch for signs of infection, stroke, and increasing anemia.
- Learn the importance of hydration and diet.
- Learn to recognize normal growth and development milestones.

2 to 6 Years
- Increase the penicillin dose to 250 mg twice a day, by mouth, and continue folic acid.
- Continue to learn about normal growth and development milestones, hydration, avoidance of over-dependence, and setting limits.
- Schedule clinic visits every three months.
- Make sure your child receives a transcranial Doppler every year for stroke prevention.

- Complete all immunizations.
- Learn about pain-management principles.
- Ask your doctor whether glutamine is suitable for your five-year-old child.
- Educate day-care workers, school nurses, and teachers about sickle cell with handouts, meetings, and letters.

PSYCHOSOCIAL ISSUES

During this period, a child goes through many miraculous changes. He or she will take that first step, begin to talk, and develop a growing sense of self as a social being. For the parents of children with sickle cell disease, these changes bring their own problems. During this period your child may become aware that his or her physical life is different from that of his or her companions. It is very important that you treat your child with sickle cell disease the same way as their siblings. It is not easy to tell a child about an illness that he or she may have for a lifetime, nor is it easy to cope with a child who is simply fed up with the demands of chronic disease and sometimes refuses to cooperate.

Talking With Your Child

Talking with a child about chronic disease should take place only in stages, according to the child's level of understanding at the time. Of course, your child will have questions. So will your other children. The best policy is to answer your children's questions simply and factually, in terms they can understand. Don't be grim or sad, but don't lie or sugar-coat the truth either. Kids will always see through our lies, however well intentioned, and a certain amount of precious trust will be lost.

What To Do When Your Child Acts Out

Any typical child will sometimes refuse to eat or do what they should and as they are told. This is especially true for anyone with a chronic disease: they will also get fed up with taking pills, seeing doctors, and being stuck with needles for blood tests. A child's resistance to treatment can be heartbreaking. It may start at an early age and usually peaks in the preteen and teen years, when some kids not only won't cooperate but deliberately do things that they know can provoke sickle cell crises—like not drinking enough water—in order to manipulate the rest of the family. Your approach to disciplining your child should be the same as if they did not have sickle cell disease.

At an early age, children learn that when they have a pain episode they get a lot of extra attention and, more often than not, get their way. Sometimes, they may resist treatment, feeling that such resistance gives them power. In general, you should not allow your child to use their disease to get special attention. They should participate in family duties and activities, attend school and church, and behave like their siblings. This will help them and reduce bad feelings between them and their siblings.

The best way to avoid these attention and power-seeking episodes is to keep the lines of communication with your child open. If you can do that, your child, should he or she choose to act out, can usually be talked back into good sense. But sometimes, even a parent's best efforts may fail. That's when family counseling may be helpful.

In general, what the child, or any person suffering a disability, wants to know is what to expect from the disease, and what to expect from the healthcare system in the way of treatment. The better the child is prepared for the pain and discomfort that the disease, and sometimes the treatment itself, may bring, the better he or she will be able to go along with it.

Your own patience and love will make themselves felt. Trust that. In the bad times, mothers, friends, other relatives, and counselors can help, as can support groups. Be willing to lean on those who will gladly help you carry the weight.

COMMON MANIFESTATIONS

Knowing what symptoms to expect prepares you to react to them. Here are signs to watch for as your child grows.

Birth to 2 Months

Babies of this age generally have no symptoms of sickle cell disease because they still have enough fetal blood to protect them against the effects of sickle hemoglobin (Hb SS).

3 to 6 Months

Symptoms of sickle cell disease often start at this age, when the baby's fetal hemoglobin is quickly being replaced by adult sickle hemoglobin. The first warning sign in the child is often a painful swelling of the fingers and toes, referred to as *hand-foot syndrome*, or *acute sickle dactylitis*. This is the result of an imbalance between the demand for and the supply of blood in these fingers and toes. Rapidly growing bone marrow chokes off its own blood supply by narrowing, or compressing, the blood vessels. In a baby with sickle cell disease, fever can be caused by a life-threatening infection, and medical care should be obtained immediately. Caregivers should know how to take the child's temperature and recognize a fever.

Signs of fever and infection in the baby include:

- extreme crankiness;
- incessant crying;
- rapid breathing;
- screaming even when touched or held by family members;
- lack of energy;
- poor appetite; and/or
- decrease in the number of wet diapers (which indicates dehydration).

In the United States and other parts of the world where malaria has been eliminated, the first episode of sickle cell pain is often brought on by bacterial infection. Where malaria is still common, the first episode may be brought on by malarial infection.

6 Months to 5 Years

For the sickle cell patient, this period of childhood is characterized by:

- a progressive breakdown of the child's red blood cells and subsequent anemia that shows itself in pallor (paleness) of the palms, soles, lips, and eyelids; and
- jaundice, or yellow discoloration of the skin and the whites of the eyes, due to the deposition of bilirubin, a pigment generated from the breakdown of hemoglobin.

COMPLICATIONS

Unfortunately, sickle cell disease can cause any of a number of secondary complications. Being familiar with them prepares you to recognize them early, know what to do, and cope with them should they develop.

Hand-Foot Syndrome

Sickle dactylitis, or hand-foot syndrome, is one of the first complications seen in sickle cell disease, usually occurring between ages six months and two years. One-third to one-half of patients may experience this complication during early childhood; it is very rare in later life.

Hand-foot syndrome is the result of blocked blood flow and damage to the small bones of the fingers and toes, which causes a rapid, painful expansion of the bone marrow cavity of these small bones. This painful swelling of the back of both hands and feet was the symptom that led to diagnosis before newborn screening became common.

Treatment of hand-foot syndrome includes hydration and pain control with acetaminophen. Bone changes occurring during episodes of dactylitis can be caused by, or mistaken for, osteomyelitis (infection in the bone).

Fever and Infections
Bacterial infections are the most common cause of death in children with sickle cell disease during the first five years of life. Those under three years of age are at greatest risk for life-threatening infections, but dangerous infections can be seen at any age. The sickle cell patient's decreased ability to fight off overwhelming infection is the result of the spleen not working properly. The spleen is the body's major defense against deadly germs. Serious infections such as blood infections (sepsis), infection surrounding the brain (meningitis), and lung infection (pneumonia) caused by these germs are common and often may be life-threatening.

The bones and joints may also become infected. Infections of the bladder and kidney are more common and may be more severe than in individuals without sickle cell disease. Lives can be saved by detecting these infections early and treating them with the proper antibiotic.

Preventive measures include the following:

- giving daily penicillin at birth until age six;
- giving pneumococcal conjugate vaccine (PCV13 or Prevnar 13), 23-valent pneumococcal polysaccharide vaccine (PPSV23 or Pneumovax), and Hemophilus influenza type B (Hib) vaccine;
- immunization for hepatitis, meningococcus, and influenza, and routine immunization for childhood diseases as recommended by the CDC's vaccine schedule;
- washing hands after bathroom breaks;
- knowing how to check for fever and learning what to do about it; and

- not eating undercooked meat, poultry, shellfish, eggs, or egg products like mayonnaise, which can allow bacteria to enter the bloodstream from the digestive system.

Be especially careful with warm-weather celebrations like picnics, barbecues, and family reunions, which can lead to steep, rapid climbs in the concentrations of bacteria like *Salmonella* and *Campylobacter* in the aforementioned types of foods because they are not constantly refrigerated. These bacteria do not necessarily make the food taste peculiar. Also, be attentive to washing fruits and vegetables carefully if they're not going to be peeled, as their outsides may harbor some of these same bacteria as well as pesticide residues. Do not cut or chop any food that will be served raw, such as fruits or vegetables, with knives or chopping boards that have been used with meat, poultry, shellfish, fish, eggs, or egg products without first washing them thoroughly with soap and hot water. Make sure meats and eggs are properly cooked to avoid infection. Remember that *Salmonella* is also a common cause of bone infections (osteomyelitis) in folks with sickle cell disease. All sickle cell patients with a fever should consider it an emergency, and consult a doctor immediately.

Splenic Sequestration

The spleen is an organ in the upper-left area of the abdomen, under the lower ribs. The spleen filters out abnormal red blood cells and helps the body's immune system fight infection. Sometimes, in persons with sickle cell disease or other hemoglobinopathies, red blood cells can be trapped in the spleen, a condition known as splenic sequestration. This is similar to bleeding internally because the blood trapped in the spleen cannot circulate to the heart or brain. This condition can range from mild to life-threatening, depending on how much of the body's red blood cells are trapped. Because splenic sequestration is a sudden trapping of unusually large amounts of blood in the spleen, the spleen enlarges rapidly. The movement of blood from general circulation into the spleen can lead to shock or circulatory collapse.

Patients experiencing this episode may show any of these signs:

- increased paleness;
- increased crying;
- rapid heartbeat (tachycardia);
- shortness of breath;

- 🩸 dizziness
- 🩸 tiredness and weakness;
- 🩸 stomach swelling—left upper area (due to the enlarging spleen); and
- 🩸 fever.

Doctors detect splenic sequestration by feeling for the enlarged spleen and testing for low red blood cell counts. You also can learn how to feel for an enlarged spleen with some training and practice. Your healthcare provider can teach this to you when you bring in your child for a checkup.

The use of a wooden tongue depressor as a "spleen measuring stick" provides an accurate way of assessing and recording spleen size at home and in the clinic. In small children, one end can be placed on the left nipple and the distance to the spleen tip recorded in ink and dated. In older children, the distance from the ribs to the spleen tip in the left nipple line is recorded. Limits can be set by drawing red lines in ink and instructing the parent to bring the child in for immediate care if the spleen is increased to the line. Parents should check the spleen size on a regular basis and whenever the child appears ill. Names and phone numbers of people who need to be contacted can be written on the back of the spleen stick. Parents should bring the spleen stick with them to every follow-up and emergency visit.

If your child is doing well, then feel for the spleen several times a week just to get practice. You should always feel for an enlarged spleen if your child:

- 🩸 looks pale, which may be a sign of blood loss. In darker-skinned people, paleness may be easier to detect by looking at the lips, the inner eyelids, and the fingernail beds. Usually these areas are red or dark pink, but if they look light pink or white, then the child is pale.
- 🩸 seems unusually tired, another sign of a low blood count.
- 🩸 is unusually cranky or irritable, and perhaps has a headache. When the red blood cell count is very low, oxygen delivery to the brain may be inadequate, causing a headache.
- 🩸 is sensitive to touch in the upper-left part of the abdomen—the area overlying the spleen.

If you suspect that your child has an enlarged spleen or is displaying any of the above symptoms, take him or her immediately for a medical evaluation. In a child with sickle cell disease, splenic sequestration can be extremely serious, and speedy evaluation and treatment may save his or her life.

Splenic sequestration may happen more than once. To prevent this, your doctor may start you on a monthly blood transfusion program or schedule surgery to remove the spleen, a procedure known as an elective splenectomy.

Strokes
BLOCKED BLOOD FLOW TO THE BRAIN

Strokes are common in children with sickle syndromes. Strokes may occur in the first year of life, and 80% occur before the age of twenty. There is a very high recurrence rate, approaching 85% in the three years after the first episode. Immediate blood transfusions may reduce the permanent damage from the stroke. Transfusion of red blood cells on a regular schedule markedly reduces the chances of new strokes. Symptoms of a new or impending stroke include:

- weakness and loss of sensation (numb feeling in the face, arms, or legs)
- dizziness, balance problems
- seizures
- slurred speech
- difficulty talking or understanding
- difficulty walking
- fainting (passing out)
- changes in vision
- unusual headache

A stroke occurs when blood flow is blocked to a part of the brain by sickled cells or by bleeding from a burst blood vessel. Stroke is an emergency requiring hospital admission, MRI or CT scans, and immediate blood transfusions. Special rehabilitation may be needed with physical and speech therapy to recover skills that may have been damaged.

More commonly, smaller strokes may cause subtle changes in the child's personality or thinking and may leave temporary or permanent function problems. In some strokes, the vessels supplying the brain are blocked for only a short time; this is called a *transient ischemic attack* or TIA. A TIA is a serious warning signal to start preventive strategies with monthly blood transfusions. This monthly treatment keeps the hemoglobin S level at less than 30%. Monthly transfusions are done by giving blood through a simple transfusion or by exchanging sickle blood with normal blood, usually with a machine. This helps prevent the first major stroke and can also help prevent future strokes if one has occurred.

You cannot stop monthly transfusions once they've started, because stopping them would make a stroke likely to occur. And remember, monthly blood transfusions cause iron overload. They mean exposure to other people's blood, which can build up to a reaction, and it also means exposure to infectious diseases. However, studies clearly show that these risks are worth taking because they prevent strokes.

Bone marrow transplantation from a human leukocyte antigen (HLA)-matched brother or sister may offer children who have had strokes the best chance for a more normal life. New types of bone marrow transplantation are being studied so that more children with strokes and other complications can benefit from this treatment, even children without HLA-matched siblings. (See Chapter 14).

Strokes in children with increased risk may be detected by transcranial Doppler (TCD) ultrasound screening. (See next section.)

Although "clot busters" such as tPA (tissue plasminogen activator) are often used in vaso-occlusive strokes that are not associated with sickle cell disease, their role in early treatment of strokes in those with sickle cell disease has not yet been tested.

In general, the medical team treats stroke victims by:

- supporting breathing and heart functions;
- preventing bedsores;
- preventing aspiration of food;
- supporting good nutrition;
- avoiding infection; and
- aggressively using physical and occupational therapy to prevent loss of joint flexibility and muscle strength, and other rehabilitation for speech, memory, or other issues.

TRANSCRANIAL DOPPLER ULTRASOUND (TCD) AND STROKE PREVENTION

Between 8% and 12% of children with sickle cell diseases Hb SS and Hb S β^0 thalassemia are at risk for having a stroke. Another 10%–15% of children could have "silent stroke"—damage to the brain that cannot be detected on physical exam.

Stroke in these children usually results from a narrowing or closure of arteries supplying blood flow to the brain. Transcranial Doppler ultrasound (TCD) is a device that uses painless sound waves to detect areas of increased blood flow in the blood vessels of the brain. When the blood vessels are narrowed due to sickle cell damage, the blood makes a louder noise as it travels faster through the narrow area. This is like the noise in a water hose when you make the hose bend. When this test detects a constriction, or narrowing, of the blood vessels, there is a greater risk of having a stroke, and further testing is necessary.

Studies have shown that transfusions markedly reduce the likelihood of the first stroke in high-risk children with positive TCD results. Annual TCD screening is recommended for all children with sickle cell disease type Hb SS and $S\beta^0$ thal between the ages of 2 and 16.

Acute Chest Pain

Children with sickle cell disease may experience chest pain as a result of:

- blocked blood flow to the lungs;
- infection;
- pneumonia;
- part of the "all over" pain of a pain episode; and/or
- sickling in the ribs.

Acute chest syndrome is chest pain, fever, difficulty breathing, and new changes in the X-ray of the lungs. It can be caused by infection (pneumonia), blocking of blood flow to the lungs, or sickling in the lungs. The person may have chest pain when he or she breathes in and out, fever, weakness, or a high white blood cell count. This medical emergency is a common cause of hospitalization.

Pain Crisis

A pain crisis is the most frequent acute symptom of sickle cell disease. While some patients may go for years without an episode, others may have an episode once or twice a month or more. Many pain crises are able to be managed at home using rest, drinking fluids, and taking oral pain medicines. Some of these may be very severe, requiring narcotic painkillers by vein and intravenous fluids.

While most pain crises may occur without an obvious trigger factor, the triggers for many pain crises are:

- overdoing it
- stress;
- fever;
- low oxygen levels;
- *acidosis* (a change in the blood chemistry to the acidic side caused by infection, exhaustion, drug reactions, or liver, kidney, or lung problems);
- chilly temperatures; and
- dehydration.

These triggers can all lead to sickling of the red blood cells, with clumping of groups of sickled cells and blockage of blood vessels. The resulting low blood flow to the target tissue causes pain.

Pain crises often involve the arms and legs as well as the head, abdomen, chest, and back, depending upon which blood vessel is being blocked. The pain episode may be extensive, causing severe bone pain and secondary infection of the bone and bone marrow.

A pain episode is commonly treated with liberal amounts of oral and/or intravenous fluids, oral or injectable pain medicines, and treatment of the triggers that caused the pain episode.

Abdominal organs may be affected during a pain crisis. Repeated damage to the spleen eventually leads to its destruction through a condition called *auto-splenectomy*. The loss of the spleen can, in turn, increase a person's risk for serious infections. This happens early in life for those with Hb SS, and later in life for those with Hb SC or Hb S beta thalassemia.

Other abdominal organs besides the spleen may be affected during pain crises. The symptoms may resemble those of appendicitis or gallbladder attacks. In fact, an abdominal pain episode and an abdominal surgical emergency can sometimes happen at the same time.

More Severe Anemia

In sickle cell patients, the presence of anemia, low hemoglobin, or a less-than-normal number of red blood cells is lifelong, starting in the first year of life as the fetal hemoglobin level falls. The average red blood cell life span is reduced from a normal 120 days to an average of 10 to 20 days. This causes the bone marrow factory to work overtime in order to make new red blood cells at a faster rate. When red blood cells break apart, the hemoglobin inside is converted to bilirubin, which can make the white part of the eyes look yellow, or jaundiced. In later childhood and early adult life, the excess bilirubin causes gallstones.

A splenic sequestration episode occurs when the sickled red blood cells become trapped in the small blood vessels inside the spleen. This is a cause of anemia (discussed in detail in the sequestration section).

When the bone marrow factory stops making new red blood cells, it is called an *aplastic episode*. It occurs most commonly during early childhood, but it can occur at any age. The person with this episode has all of the symptoms of having fewer red blood cells, including increasing tiredness, weakness, shortness of breath, dizziness upon standing, and increasing paleness.

Treatment of an aplastic episode usually requires a blood transfusion. If the cause of the infection is bacterial, antibiotic therapy may be indicated as well.

There can also be increased destruction of the red blood cells during pain crisis and with infection. This is called a hemolytic episode and it is treated in the same manner as an aplastic episode, with blood transfusion, fluids, and treatment of any infection.

PREVENTIVE MEASURES

Penicillin

Because infections are among the greatest dangers to those with sickle cell disease, all children from birth until age six should be given daily penicillin. The low dose of penicillin is not enough antibiotic to rid the body of an invading infection, but it helps the body to defend itself until you can get the child to a medical facility for more powerful antibiotics. The usual penicillin dose for newborns until age two is 125 mg twice a day as a liquid. At age two, the dose goes up to 250 mg twice a day. This simple low-dose penicillin treatment has saved many patients' lives. Liquid penicillin must be refrigerated and replaced every two weeks if not used.

If your child becomes allergic to penicillin, there are other effective antibiotics. Discuss these with your child's physician and follow their recommendations.

Vaccination

Children with sickle cell disease should have all of the immunizations that are recommended for other children. Immunizations help the body build natural defenses against invading germs and viruses. The pneumococcal polyvalent vaccine Prevnar 13 is a breakthrough that gives protection from birth through the vulnerable early childhood period. Vaccination, plus daily penicillin, will reduce the chance that a fatal pneumococcal infection will occur. It is not a guarantee, so parents must be on the watch for signs of infection, mainly fever. Do not continue to give acetaminophen or NSAIDs longer than the recommended time after vaccination. Seek medical care if fever or irritability persists.

Because vaccines and schedules may change, the CDC website (*www.cdc.gov/vaccines/schedules*) has the most reliable and up-to-date information. Patients and parents should review all the recommendations with their care providers.

Incentive Spirometry

Incentive spirometers, or blow bottles, should be used by the child during any pain episode or event that causes bed rest. The blow bottle is a way to keep the lungs' air sacks open and allow oxygen to get to the red blood cells. Using the blow bottle can help prevent acute chest syndrome.

Hydroxyurea and Glutamine as Preventive Treatment

Please see Chapters 5 and 13 for the benefits and risks of these two FDA-approved preventive treatments.

Bone Marrow Transplantation

Bone marrow transplantation may be considered if a child with sickle cell disease experiences dangerous complications like stroke, acute chest syndrome, or frequent pain episodes. The child ideally should have an human leukocyte antigen (HLA)-matched donation from a brother or sister; however, use of other donors who are only a partial match (not an exact match) is being studied. Successful bone marrow transplant has cured sickle cell disease in over 1,600 children worldwide. Some now believe that any child with symptoms and a matched sibling donor should be considered for this curative therapy. The procedure has a risk of death in less than 5% of those going through it. The procedure takes several months and costs nearly $300,000. A full description of bone marrow transplant is in Chapter 14.

5

Six to Twelve Years

By the age of six, your child's routines and procedures described in the previous chapter will be established. But some new symptoms will appear, and some of the old ones will become more pronounced. You will have new tasks to do, such as monitoring your child's medical condition and helping your child keep up good preventive practices.

Also during this period, your child will start school, and you will want to have a clear understanding with his or her teachers and other school staff members about the special requirements your child may have. You should consider developing an Individualized Education Plan (IEP) and may need a 504 Plan (discussed below).

In this chapter we will talk about these new issues.

CLINICAL ISSUES

- Talk with your child's doctor about stopping penicillin.
- Schedule clinic visits every four to six months.
- Start scheduling full eye examinations every year.
- Identify gallstones with an ultrasound test.
- Have your child screened for hearing loss and pulmonary function (breathing).
- Have urine screening for protein, a sign that the kidneys may be having difficulty.

PSYCHOSOCIAL AND PARENTING ISSUES

- Stress academic achievement, prevention of complications, and health maintenance.
- Begin sex education.

- Keep track of your child's psychosocial development.
- Be prepared for delayed puberty.
- Start discussions about sexuality as the questions arise. Children are being exposed to sexuality early and continuously from the media, Internet, and their friends. Parents need to be open to their children, honest, and set a good example. (See the next chapter.)
- Set limits for behavior.
- Encourage good school performance.
- Be sure you and your child keep doctors' appointments.
- Do not let sickle cell rule the house.
- Spend quality time together doing fun and memorable activities.
- Allow normal activities, keeping in mind FARMS prevention.
- Try not to favor the child with sickle cell disease over other brothers and sisters, giving all of your children quality time, responsibilities, and discipline as needed. There may be episodes of hospitalization during which the normal daily routine is disrupted. Let the other children know what is going on, and let them be involved as much as possible.

SICK ROLE

Give your child care and compassion, both when the child is well and pain free as well as when ill and in pain, with equal amounts for all of your children. Avoid making a big fuss and "rewarding" the child in times of pain and illness. Some children, and even adults, who are rewarded with attention only when they are ill or in pain develop a "sick role," using pain in order to gain attention. Your aim should be to motivate the child to get better and to continue with the daily routines of school, friends, and activities.

CAMP

Many sickle cell foundations and clinics sponsor a sickle cell camp during the summer for children six to twelve years old. These camps allow the children to have fun with other kids with sickle cell disease in a medically supervised environment. These camps usually have adult sickle cell patients as counselors to help mentor the younger patients. Check with the sickle cell community group and clinic near you to see if a camp is offered. Also check with the SeriousFun Children's Network, which has camp sessions for children with sickle cell.

AGE-SPECIFIC SYMPTOMS

- The inability of the kidneys to concentrate urine will become more obvious. Affected children will urinate more often, and persistent bed-wetting (*enuresis*) may occur. These problems understandably lead to difficulties in the child's socialization. Normal activities like camp, sleepovers, school trips, and even sitting through classes become potentially embarrassing for the child. Bed-wetting may become a source of conflict between the parent and the child if the parents do not understand the cause.
- More severe anemia may develop. This is caused by early red blood cell breakdown (*hemolysis*). This breakdown releases hemoglobin into the blood stream, where it is converted to bilirubin. Bilirubin causes the white part of the eye to turn yellow (*jaundice*). This is a very distressing symptom for children and can be a source of teasing by other children.
- The spleen can be regarded as a filter for broken red blood cells, removing them from the circulation. As a result of removing the damaged cells from the blood stream of those with sickle cell disease, the spleen enlarges. Occasionally, this organ experiences splenic sequestration, with large volumes of blood pooling within the spleen. These two processes combine to produce enlargement of the spleen.
- Your child will have an increased need for calories and energy to build new red blood cells and repair damaged tissue.
- Abnormal development of the jaw and/or breastbone occurs in some individuals. The bone marrow expands as it tries to accommodate the need for increased red blood cell production, most often in the jaws and the breastbone. Prominence of the forehead (known as *frontal bossing*), and protrusion of the jaw (known as *prognathism*) are among the abnormal bony symptoms of some people with sickle cell disease. Because the jaw protrudes, dental abnormalities and gum disease may occur more often in these children.
- Any decreased performance in school work may signal that your child is having silent strokes. Have your doctor order magnetic resonance imaging (MRI) of the brain and psychological testing.

COMPLICATIONS

New secondary problems can develop in children with sickle cell disease during this period.

Gallstones

The gallbladder holds bile, a substance made from bilirubin, the by-product of hemoglobin recycling. Bile helps your body digest fatty foods. Because of the increased red cell hemolysis in sickle cell disease, bilirubin production is increased, and this causes gallstones to form in the gallbladder.

Gallstones can cause the gallbladder to become plugged and swollen. This causes pain in the upper-right area of the stomach; other symptoms include nausea and vomiting. These symptoms can happen especially after eating fatty or fried foods.

If necessary, the gallbladder can be surgically removed.

Delayed Growth

Children with sickle cell may weigh less than others of the same age, though this varies from child to child. Older children and adolescents with sickle cell disease, on average, are shorter than their peers, but this difference disappears in adulthood. Puberty may come later in both males and females with sickle cell disease. Factors contributing to the delay include the low red blood cell count and the type of sickle cell disease the child has. In general, it is better for the individual with sickle cell disease to not be overweight, so good nutrition and not overeating should be stressed.

Treatment for delayed growth includes good general nutrition, vitamins, increased calories, and, on the psychological side, reassurance that normal maturation will occur.

Priapism

Priapism is the painful erection of the penis caused by sickling red blood cells blocking blood flow out of the penis. Priapism usually occurs between the ages of 5 and 35. It often occurs as a severe, long episode requiring hospitalization and follows multiple episodes of short duration, termed "stuttering." Episodes usually come from normal nighttime erections. Priapism may also come from a bladder infection, having sexual intercourse, or masturbation.

Treatment for priapism includes emptying the bladder, pain relief, medication that opens closed blood vessels, hydration, and blood transfusion;

surgery may be required. Impotence is a long-term consequence of repeated episodes in one-third to one-half of the cases.

Kidney Problems: Bed-Wetting, Protein
The kidney has just the right conditions—low oxygen, high salt concentration, and high acid concentration—to cause red cells to sickle. The kidney is the main filter of the blood, saving or releasing water, salts, and waste products. If early damage impairs the kidney's ability to hold on to water, large amounts of water come out in the urine, even when the body is dehydrated.

When the kidney releases too much water, children may need frequent bathroom breaks. This is important to discuss with teachers and caregivers. To help control the bed-wetting problem, use an alarm that sounds when dampness is detected. These are available at most drug stores. Encourage your child to stop drinking fluids one hour before going to bed, and make sure they go to the bathroom just before they go to bed.

Over time, damage to the kidney filters can cause protein to leak into the urine. This may be the first sign that more damage is occurring. A special urine test for protein, with data collected over 24 hours, can help predict the level of damage that is occurring. There is research underway to test preventive medications that may slow this kidney damage.

PREVENTION MEASURES

- Again, the best strategy for prevention is FARMS, as outlined in Chapter 2.
- Be sure that when your child exercises or works outdoors, he or she wears the proper clothing for the season, carries a water bottle, and drinks plenty of water. He or she must take frequent rest and water breaks.
- Your child should avoid swimming pools that are too cold or hot tubs that are too hot. Even when swimming in a warm pool, he or she should dry off immediately when getting out of the water to prevent chilling that may cause a pain episode.
- Your child should avoid emotional stress by pacing projects and work, and by avoiding situations likely to be upsetting.
- Parents and child should belong to a support group. Check with local community-based sickle cell organizations for sickle cell specific support groups. According to your beliefs, a church or faith-

- based group may offer general spiritual and emotional support.
- 🩸 Transcranial Doppler ultrasound testing should continue annually until age 16 for children with Hb SS and Hb Sβ^0 thalassemia. See Chapter 4 for further information on this test as a means of stroke prevention.

HYDROXYUREA

The effectiveness and safety of hydroxyurea was established in adults in the late 1990s for adults with sickle cell disease. Studies in even very young children show that the drug is equally safe and effective in preventing complications. Several studies suggest that sickle cell patients taking hydroxyurea are living longer than those who are not on the drug. Hydroxyurea is now accepted therapy for sickle cell patients of all ages. Nonetheless, the treatment has been used relatively less among pediatric patients. It is more common among teenagers, and most common among adults. However, in August 2018, Medunik USA announced the availability of Siklos, the first hydroxyurea-based treatment made specifically for children with sickle cell disease. This new drug could lead to an increase in the use of hydroxyurea in pediatric patients. While there is still much to be learned about hydroxyurea therapy for sickle cell patients, we know this:

- 🩸 Hydroxyurea treatment seems to improve pain; reduce anemia; and prevent acute chest syndrome, priapism, and abnormal red blood cell stickiness to the blood vessel wall (endothelium).
- 🩸 Hydroxyurea decreases the frequency of pain episodes, though it may not completely eliminate them.
- 🩸 Small studies have shown no impact of hydroxyurea on sickle cell damage to the spleen and, perhaps, no impact in avascular necrosis of bones such as the hip and shoulder joints.

Hydroxyurea prolongs life. New information indicates that the side effects for children on hydroxyurea appear to be the same as the effects for adult patients.

Potential side effects of long-term hydroxyurea therapy

COMMON

- 🩸 *Suppression of blood cell production.* Mild slowing of the rate at which new red blood cells are made is an intended effect of hydroxyurea. Hydroxyurea also slows the bone marrow's production of white blood cells and platelets. The amount of hydroxyurea taken daily needs to be carefully adjusted, and blood cell counts should be monitored every two to four weeks to make sure that the number of new red cells, white cells, and platelets do not get too low. If the white blood cells are too low, chances of infections increase. Platelet counts that are too low lead to increased chances of bleeding. Usually hydroxyurea increases the hemoglobin level because the red blood cells survive longer. Too high a dose can lower the hemoglobin, causing fatigue and problems for heart and lung function.

- *Mild nausea or upset stomach.* Most patients have this only for the first few weeks at a certain dose, then the nausea goes away. Sometimes nausea is less troublesome if the hydroxyurea is taken at bedtime.

LESS COMMON
- thinning of hair;
- darkening of skin and nails; and
- abnormal sperm counts or sperm movement.

RARE
- decreased kidney or liver function;
- dizziness; and
- changes in mood or thought.

All of these effects are expected to be reversible when the hydroxyurea is stopped. Generally, the medication can then be restarted and adjusted to a lower dose.

Leukemia—No Longer a Worry
Important new data shows that people on hydroxyurea for the treatment of sickle cell and other blood disorders do NOT have an increased rate of developing leukemia (cancer of white blood cells).

Birth Defects
It is recommended that hydroxyurea not be given to pregnant women , especially in the first two trimesters of pregnancy. Hydroxyurea should be stopped at least six weeks before conceiving a baby to help avoid the chance of birth defects. However, worry about the possibility of birth defects leads most doctors to give hydroxyurea only when individuals of reproductive age are on good contraception.

Males or females on hydroxyurea should abstain from sex or use excellent contraception. So far, the handfuls of babies born to mothers on hydroxyurea for sickle cell have not had birth defects.

Reduced Sperm Count in Males
Males taking hydroxyurea have reduced sperm counts and may have increased normal-looking sperm. This also occurs in individuals with sickle cell disease not taking hydroxyurea, so it is not clear how much is caused by the drug. Stopping hydroxyurea usually results in improved counts. Many males father children while taking hydroxyurea. It is recommended that the drug be stopped six weeks before fathering a child.

Growth and Development Problems
Some people worried that hydroxyurea treatment will slow the growth or development of children with sickle cell disease. A few years of tracking hundreds of children have not revealed growth and development problems so far, but longer study is needed. Recent studies done in young children suggest that hydroxyurea may prevent some problems with intellectual development caused by anemia and silent strokes.

Hydroxyurea Therapy in a Nutshell
Treatment with hydroxyurea has been shown to be very beneficial for individuals with Hb SS and Hb Sβ^0 thalassemia. It is now recommended that all individuals with these types of sickle cell disease consider taking hydroxyurea, and that it be offered to patients as young as nine months of age. There is no data suggesting it will benefit those with Hb SC and only a little data to support its use in Hb Sβ^+ thalassemia. Hydroxyurea therapy for a child or adult with sickle cell disease appears safe if the blood counts and other laboratory tests are monitored regularly. There are several known risks that appear to be mild and go away when the drug is stopped. Long-term side effects will not be known until we have done more research into sickle cell hydroxyurea treatment.

We strongly recommend individual discussions with your child's hematologist about the risks and benefits of hydroxyurea treatment. At Grady Hospital, we generally have two or three sessions with patients in order to:

- review the child's medical history and present condition;
- discuss individualized risks and benefits;
- provide reading material on these risks and benefits; and

🩸 draw a panel of baseline lab tests (blood counts; vitamin B12 and folate levels; kidney and liver function; testing for hepatitis, HIV infection, and pregnancy).

You need to have a doctor who will follow your child very closely for blood counts and monitor for hydroxyurea-related or other sickle cell problems.

Glutamine

Glutamine is a new medication for treating sickle cell disease that entered the US market in 2018. It works to lessen the symptoms of sickle cell disease by boosting the antioxidant properties of red blood cells. For more information on glutamine, see chapter 13.

Alternative Treatments

Besides managing the complications of sickle cell disease as they occur, the only other current alternatives to hydroxyurea or glutamine therapy are regular transfusions and bone marrow transplantation (You will find a detailed review of bone marrow transplantation in Chapter 14.).

Both of these alternatives have major risks as well as major benefits that are greater than those of hydroxyurea. Talk with your doctor about the risk/benefit balance for you or your child.

There is a large number of new treatments for sickle cell disease are in the research pipeline, but some are likely to be available outside of a clinical research trial by 2020.

GUIDE FOR TEACHERS

It is a good idea to meet with your child's teachers and find out what they know about sickle cell disease. If there is a school nurse, let him or her know about your child. Most sickle cell clinics have a handout to give teachers. You can also help educate your teachers. Here is a sample guide you can modify to your special needs.

Sample Classroom Guide

➡ Sickle cell patients may be absent because of severe pain episodes caused by the blockage of blood flow to body organs or bones, as well as other complications. These episodes may be

treated at home or could require treatment in a hospital setting. Make-up work for students should be provided to keep the student current with assignments. A hospital- or home-based teacher may be required for prolonged complications.
- Pain episodes may be prevented by allowing persons with sickle cell disease to keep well hydrated with water. Let them keep a water bottle with them or allow frequent water breaks. They will also require frequent bathroom breaks, because their kidneys cannot retain water as well as normal kidneys.
- Pain episodes may also be prevented by not allowing the individual to become overheated or exposed to cold temperatures.
- Because of their anemia, individuals with sickle cell may tire before others. Rest periods may be appropriate. Encourage physical activity, but allow them to stop and take breaks without undue attention.
- Sickle cell disease is a lifelong illness that may have various effects that can impair academic performance. These should be identified and addressed, as they would for any child. Academic performance is especially important now that life expectancy for those with sickle cell has increased dramatically and they need preparation for vocations that are not physically demanding. Those with sickle cell, like anyone, can become professionals like doctors, engineers, and lawyers.
- Most children with sickle cell disease should have an IEP.
- Sickle cell patients may have a yellow tint to their eyes because of the increased bilirubin from red cell breakdown, but, this is not usually a liver problem. They also may have a shorter stature and delayed puberty because of the anemia.
- Students with sickle cell should be treated as normally as possible, with awareness that they may have intermittent episodes of pain, infection, or fatigue.
- Learn about sickle cell, and understand the challenges that students with this disease must face.
- Have a plan of action with the individual to do what you can to keep him or her productive and complication-free.

Medical attention is needed when any of the following occur:

- fever;
- headache;
- chest pain;
- abdominal pain; or
- numbness or weakness.

A mild pain episode may be managed with increased fluid intake and a non-narcotic pain pill like ibuprofen or acetaminophen.

Your school can launch a sickle cell awareness program by encouraging activities like these:

- Invite a speaker from your local sickle cell foundation or clinic to educate the entire class or staff about sickle cell.
- Become involved in public awareness events like walks, fun runs, kids' camp, and fundraisers.
- Encourage blood donations and blood drives in your community. Many with sickle cell need transfusions to prevent childhood strokes and other complications.
- Support sickle cell research to provide new treatments.
- Encourage sickle cell patients to be the best they can be.

Disabled School Children and the Law

An important law to consider is the Individuals with Disabilities Act (IDEA), PL 101-476, which states the rights of children with disabilities, and those of their parents. A basic part of the law is the right of parents to help decide about their child's education. IDEA says, "States must provide a free appropriate public education to all students (ages 3–21) who are disabled. Children must be assessed for their disabilities, strengths, and needs."

Another important law to keep in mind is PL 93-112, the Rehabilitation Act, Section 504, which was designed to end discrimination on the basis of a physical or mental disability in any program getting federal financial aid—including public schools. Some children with health problems may not need, or be eligible for, services under IDEA, but they may need special help or modifications under Section 504. Some examples of modifications may include a shortened school day/week, special equipment, and modified academic coursework.

Hospital/Homebound Services: This is a plan for children in kindergarten through 12th grade who have missed school at least 10 days due to illness, and who may miss more. A teacher is sent by the school system to the home for at least three hours a week.

What Parents Can Do

- Become active in your child's school. Get to know the teachers and school staff, and maintain open communication.
- Be very clear about what you want for your child. Tell teachers about your child's illness. Let teachers know how to meet your child's school needs. Tell them what you know about your child's physical problems. For example, your child may have a hard time carrying books or have problems keeping up in gym when sickle cell problems occur. Also tell the school staff to be alert to the signs of sickle cell difficulties, such as fatigue, fever, and jaundice.
- Keep in mind that if your child needs to be in the hospital, he or she may use the hospital's school program. You can help by bringing your child's homework to the hospital's teachers so that your child may continue to receive school credit. Being a part of the hospital's school program also helps to decrease the pressure on your child by helping him or her keep up with schoolmates.
- Ask school staff members to share their observations of your child with you.
- Keep a good relationship with the school staff.
- Attend all meetings that are held, such as parent/teacher conferences and IEP meetings. Bring a friend or family member with you who knows your child. Take notes, and don't be afraid to ask for time to think about a certain decision.

- It is important for you to understand your child's illness. The disease may cause depression, withdrawal, sleeping too much or not enough, acting out, or changes in eating patterns in your child. If any of these things happen, it would help to speak to a mental health professional for your child and possibly for the entire family. It is important to seek help to deal with the pressures involved with a child with sickle cell disease. Keep track of your child's progress. Is the plan you agreed on working? Do any changes need to be made? Check in with the teacher often to see how things are going. Keep a notebook to give and receive information.

- Be aware of the needs of all of your children. They may feel anxious, angry, or depressed. A sibling may feel guilty because he or she is healthy. They may feel jealous, lonely, withdrawn, or that they are not being treated fairly because the child with sickle cell disease is getting a lot of attention, especially during periods of pain crisis or when in the hospital.

- Sickle cell disease may affect learning in some children. If there is concern about a child's ability to learn, discuss this with your physician as soon as possible. If a child has had a history of strokes or is having trouble with learning or behavior, it may be necessary for him or her to receive psychological testing to determine ability to learn.

- Children with sickle cell disease may be absent from school a lot due to clinic visits, pain crises, or other health problems. Make sure classwork and homework assignments are available to you to keep the student from falling behind. If your child is in the hospital, communicate with the child's teachers and give them his or her classwork. If necessary, arrange tutoring for your student.

- Keep in mind that children with sickle cell disease tire more easily than other children. *This is important for the physical education teacher to understand.* These children should be given the time to rest when needed. Physical activity is an important part of good health, so it is best to include them even if they are hesitant to join in. If you prefer that your child be excused from any activity, permission should be granted.

6

The Teen Years: Thirteen to Eighteen

HEIDY'S STORY

For as long as I can remember, I have longed to be normal, and sometimes that longing made my life even harder than it was already. I was ashamed to be ill, and sometimes angry that pain episodes and other medical problems kept me from living what, to me, seemed the free and easy lives of my friends.

But when I was ten, in the hospital for treatment for one of my many pain episodes, something clicked. I sat up in bed and told myself I'd never feel sorry for myself again.

The way I remember coming to that insight and resolution was this. I'd been hospitalized more than 100 times for pain episodes. I understood what caused the pain, but that didn't make the trips to the emergency room any easier. I knew the treatment. Strong drugs like morphine and Demerol and fluid given to me intravenously.

I hated the trips to the emergency room, even though without them I couldn't get rid of the pain. Sometimes the pain was okay, but sometimes I felt as if I were about to die. Month after month, I'd have one of these crises, and I'd pray to God for an answer to the question I never stopped asking: "Why me?"

Sometimes, when I was a child, I'd ignore the limits the doctors had warned me about. I'd swim in the school pool, even though I'd sometimes get sick afterwards because the water was too cold. I was trying very hard to kid myself. I actually believed for a while that if I didn't think of myself as being sick I wouldn't be, so I ignored many warnings and tried hard to hide my sickness from friends and family.

That went on for years, and during that time I wasn't doing very well as a patient. When I was older and a little more open to reason, my doctors told me that I would be able to deal with sickle cell disease only if I learned about it. So I did learn. As I got older, I understood that sometimes I had to deal with doctors and nurses who didn't know much about sickle cell disease. I made it my business to educate them by telling them patiently about the illness and about what I needed to make my symptoms more manageable. I began to follow the research and know about the people and clinics searching for a cure. To sum it all up, as a child I was afraid to tell the truth about who I really was. I was afraid even to know that truth myself. Now I accept it, and I let other people know because I realize that sickle cell disease is part of me.

Today I can honestly say that, in a way, sickle cell has become a blessing. It has made me stronger by making me come to terms with myself. I know I'm one of the lucky ones. There are some people out there with this disease who lack the help they need. I have a loving and understanding family. Even though they cannot feel my pain, they are with me every step of the way. As for friends, they come and go, but there are some I have had since childhood who cry every time they see me in pain. I am thankful for them. My quest for normalcy has faded into a devotion to aid, as much as I can, those with my disease. I am now at the beginning of a new quest to find a cure for my disease.

* * *

COMMON MANIFESTATIONS

As Heidy could tell you, each stage of maturation brings new problems and the need for new solutions. Adolescence can be hard on anyone, but it is especially hard on people with sickle cell disease. A broad range of physical ailments can, and do, occur. The issues discussed in previous chapters may occur, but we won't cover them here. Instead, we'll focus on changes in this age group.

Pain Episodes

It is not uncommon for pain episodes to increase in frequency and severity during the teenage years. Prevention and treatment is similar to that outlined in Chapter 4. Females may have pain with each menstrual period. Like Heidy, many in this age group try and ignore their disease and be "normal," and this may contribute to complications.

Bone Disease

It is thought that much of the pain that occurs during an acute pain episode is caused by reduced blood flow to bones due to sickling. If the blockage is prolonged, the bone is damaged; this is called a bone infarction. Bone infarcts heal over time, but it often takes longer for the pain to resolve. Areas where there is bone infarction are tender to the touch may have swelling and redness over the damaged area, and this can be confused with bone infections. They are self-limited and heal without persistent problems.

Many individuals with sickle cell disease are vitamin D deficient, and this may contribute to pain and bone damage. Vitamin D levels should be monitored and deficiency treated with vitamin D supplementation.

The hips and shoulders have relatively poor blood flow, and sickling can cause damage to the bone that results in collapse of the shoulder and hip bones. This causes chronic pain and decreases movement. It can be progressive and may require surgery to replace the joints.

Chronic Bone Infections

Chronic bone infections are all too common. These bone infections (known as osteomyelitis) are difficult to cure. Sometimes they require months of intravenous and/or oral antibiotic therapy, often combined with localized surgery. X-rays, bone scans, and gallium scans (a type of imaging) are helpful in suspected cases of osteomyelitis. Definitive diagnosis usually requires biopsy, with culture, to identify the infection and determine which antibiotics will work the best.

Priapism

In males with sickle cell diseases, priapism, or painful prolonged erections of the penis, may occur as a result of sickled cells blocking the outflow of blood from the penis. Repeated episodes of priapism can, unfortunately, lead to erectile dysfunction and permanent impotence. Young males with priapism may try and hide the problem. Treatment is with hydration, pain control, and warm baths at home. If priapism does not respond to these, treatment in the emergency room is needed where more intense pain control and hydration can be given. Irrigation of the shaft of the penis with fluids to flush out sickled cells and inject drugs to increase blood flow may be needed. Prolonged and repeated episodes may require surgical shunts. Clinical trials are beginning to study better ways to treat priapism. Although none have been well studied in clinical trials, medications used to prevent priapism include hydroxyurea, pseudoephedrine, etilefrine, terbutaline, and sildenafil.

Chronic Leg Ulcers
Chronic ulcers may form, especially on or near the inner side of the ankles. They result from blockage of the blood supply to the skin by sickled red blood cells and other material. The ulcers generally appear pale, with a yellowish tinge. More details about leg ulcers are in the next chapter.

Delayed Puberty
Puberty in children with sickle cell disease is sometimes delayed, as it is in children with other debilitating, chronic illnesses. For girls, the onset of the first menstrual period (or *menarche*) and breast development may both be late. In boys, the testicles remain small longer, and body hair growth may be delayed. Puberty will eventually come, but the delay may have significant impact on self-esteem.

Emotional Problems
Studies show that sickle cell youth are very well adjusted considering the seriousness of their disease and its impact on their lives. However, emotional problems can result from trying to deal with the overwhelming range of problems including fatigue, bouts of acute illness, pain, fear of death, death of friends with sickle cell, and social isolation. Depression is common but can be treated by professional counselors and antidepressant medications. School grades can fall. Drug abuse may occur as a way of coping with physical and emotional pain. Adolescence is a difficult time for the individual and their families, even in the absence of sickle cell disease. All of the challenges faced by those without sickle cell will also be experienced by the individuals with sickle cell disease, with the added burden of frequent illness, delayed puberty, and difficulty participating in some peer activities like sports.

PREVENTIVE MEASURES

Patients and parents will already be familiar with the best ways to prevent pain—a set of guidelines known as FARMS. See Chapter 2 for a discussion of these guidelines.

No Smoking, No Alcohol, No Street Drugs
Smoking can cause damage to the lungs that will rob the red blood cells of oxygen increasing sickling and may contribute to pulmonary hypertension later in life. Nicotine causes blood vessels to narrow and may add to problems

in blood flow caused by sickling. Alcohol dehydrates the body and can damage the liver over time. Alcohol can also make the blood more acidic, and this can cause sickling. Finally, alcohol impairs judgment and can lead to mistakes. Most of our older adults report that they will predictably end up in the emergency room with a pain crisis the day after consuming too much alcohol.

Illegal drugs like cocaine also predictably cause episodes of pain. They can kill people who don't have sickle cell disease and are even more dangerous for those with it. It is also important to point out that because they are illegal, possession and use of these drugs can lead to time in jail, a very hostile place for someone with sickle cell disease.

Sexuality and Birth Control Options

Children and youth are getting massive exposure to sex from friends, on the Internet, and in the media at a very early age. Parents need to be open, honest, truthful, and available to their children so they can provide factual information and moral guidance for their children. Children need to be prepared to deal with the normal changes in their bodies during puberty. They also need to be prepared to handle the depiction of irresponsible sexual behaviors in popular media, the promotion of sex in advertising, and intense peer pressure.

Discussions should include not only the facts about sex, but also the benefits and consequences of behaviors while expressing sexuality. Parents need to set good examples in their choices, and their children should be instilled with a sense of responsibility, trusted to make the right decisions, and supported through their choices.

Individuals with sickle cell disease may face additional challenges because of the desire to fit in and "be normal." Delayed puberty and small stature at this age can lead to a poor self-image and make them more vulnerable to peer pressure. Engaging in sexual activity at this early age may have more consequences if they have a child or contract a sexually transmitted disease (STD).

The only safe way to avoid these consequences is to just say no and delay sex until later, in the context of a stable, monogamous relationship. More youths are choosing this course and need to be supported in this choice.

Parents should counsel teens about the benefits of abstinence and monogamous relationships. There are a number of good resources on parenting than contain guidance about this sensitive area.

If a teen is sexually active, they need a complete and accurate education about birth control and the prevention of sexually transmitted diseases. Parents should be willing to provide this information or connect their child with health professionals who can. Prevention against HIV and other sexually transmitted diseases that can ruin their lives is critical. For a female with sickle cell disease, enduring pregnancy and parenting a baby requires a robust support system that is often not present for a single mother. Males with sickle cell disease may have great difficulty with the demands of supporting a child while they are trying to complete their education and preparing for a vocation.

Birth Control Options to Consider
- The combination of a latex condom and spermicidal foam provides safe, effective contraception and is *the only method* that may reduce the transmission of AIDS and other STDs. The condom should be put on before any penetration occurs.
- Oral contraception is probably the most effective method for preventing pregnancy, but provides no protection from STDs. Oral contraceptives are probably safe if progesterone-only preparations are used, but they may present a higher risk of complications if a teenager is a smoker, is overweight or obese, has had blood clots, or has a disease with increased clotting, such as lupus. Consultation with a gynecologist who is comfortable treating individuals with sickle cell disease is essential for counseling on birth control.
- The intrauterine device (IUD) is also effective, though with this form of contraception there is increased risk of infection. Again, STDs are not prevented.
- Diaphragms are usually less effective, but may be satisfactory if combined with a spermicidal preparation. They may provide some STD protection.
- Progestin-only-based prevention by pill, or by injection preparations such as Depo-Provera, is also effective. They may also reduce menstrual-associated pain crisis. But please note that progestin-only-based contraception may result in unpredictable bleeding. It may also increase LDL or "bad" cholesterol and decrease HDL, the "good" cholesterol. It may also increase triglycerides and blood pressure.

- Even with the most careful precautions, a sexually active teen may become a mother or a father, so it is vital for your child to consider the potential for passing sickle cell disease or trait on to his or her own child. If he or she is involved with a partner, strongly urge the couple to undergo genetic counseling *before* becoming intimate. Remember that sickle cell diseases are 100% preventable!

Caution: *It is critically important to know that oral contraception, IUDs, diaphragms, or progesterone will not protect you against HIV/AIDS.*

CLINICAL ISSUES

- Discuss sexual development and related issues with you child.
- Assist your child in progressing to independence by stressing self-management, coping skills, and academic achievement.
- Discuss with your child birth control, prevention of complications, learning physical limits, sexually transmitted diseases, and substance abuse.
- Provide peer support by encouraging support group contact and activities.
- Discuss realistic job and career goals and education beyond high school.
- Schedule clinic visits every four to six months.
- Teens should have a screening test to detect protein in the urine. This may be the first warning about kidney damage.
- Immunization against human papilloma virus is recommended for girls in order to prevent cervical cancer.

PSYCHOSOCIAL ISSUES FOR TEENS

Adolescence has always been a challenge for teens, and modern social changes have increased this challenge for all teens. Teens want to be accepted by their peers, and their disease may increase their chances of rejection and teasing. The disease may interfere with developing friendships because they miss social opportunities and ability to participate in sports. Parents should open their home to friends and provide teens with constructive guidance on relating to their friends. Participation in church, clubs, and support groups should be encouraged.

Teens need to be prepared for independence. A gradual increase in responsibility for management of their medications, appointments, refills, and health habits should be instituted early. This requires a positive approach and willingness to allow them to make mistakes.

Pushing one's limits and risk taking is almost universal during adolescence. Teens should be counseled about the serious dangers facing all teens. However, teens with sickle cell disease may be at higher risk of injury or death from guns, auto accidents, suicide, drugs, and alcohol than from their disease. Encourage seat belt use, avoidance of alcohol, and avoiding situations where they may be exposed to drugs or violence. Risky sexual behavior can lead to unwanted pregnancies, HIV, and other sexually transmitted diseases. It is important to spend time with teens affirming and supporting them. Supportive friends and parents can be positive influences and should serve as positive role models.

Explore the symptoms of depression or drug abuse, including sleep disturbances, eating disorders, lack of interest in favorite activities, and withdrawal from friends and family. Ask about suicidal thoughts and plans. These should be taken very seriously and professional help sought immediately if such plans are revealed.

Puberty

Increased challenges with social and psychological challenges are often increased because puberty may be delayed by two to three years in those with sickle cell disease. Teens and parents should be assured that puberty will occur. Self-esteem may suffer when one's peers are growing and developing secondary sex characteristics, and you are doing so at a much slower rate. Parents should actively teach social skills to their teens to help them deal with the stress of being different. With the onset of puberty comes emotional highs and lows. Parents need to be patience, supportive, available, and consistent though this period.

TRANSITION TO ADULT HEALTHCARE

Transition from pediatric- to adult-centered care is a major challenge for youth with sickle cell disease. In pediatrics, parents and providers are responsible for the child's care. In adulthood, the goal is for the individual to take complete responsibility of their care with the input and guidance of health professionals. Youth, parents, and healthcare professionals all must transition together through this process. It is very important to start early and develop an orderly increase in the youth's responsibility for their care. There are several excellent resources available to assist with this planning such as Got Transition (*www.GotTransition.org*) and Florida Health and Transition Services (*www.FloridaHATS.org*). There are six key elements developed by Got Transition for health professionals that individuals and families should embrace.

This process should begin at 12 years of age and continue through transfer by age 21 to 26, depending on policy and the youth's stage of development. Parents should also begin the transition of responsibility as soon as the child is developmentally ready. It is good to start with health behaviors and medications. Responsibility for talking to the doctor, refilling prescriptions, making appointments, and becoming knowledgeable about one's disease can be added as the youth becomes ready.

> **GOT TRANSITION CORE ELEMENTS**
>
> → Make youth and family aware of the transition policy
>
> → Initiate health care transition planning
>
> → Prepare youth and parents for adult model of care and discuss transfer
>
> → Transition to adult model of care
>
> → Transfer care to adult medical home and/or specialists with transfer package
>
> → Integrate young adults into adult care
>
> *Adapted from www.GotTransition.org*

The treatment philosophy in a children's hospital is quite different from that of an adult health system. Take time to get to know the adult doctors, nurses, and social workers. Learn about all of the adult services available. Many centers offer teen clinics to meet the special needs of adolescents. Teens should practice talking to the doctors and nurses about their own health history and healthcare while still accompanied by their families so they get the most out of their visits. They should also start seeing their doctors, nurses, and other healthcare professionals without their parents in the room. The following points will help teens prepare for appointments:[1]

- Do you have any new problems or questions? Write them down before the visit so you can make sure to bring them up.
- Collect your insurance information and other medical papers.

---

1 Adapted from the American Society of Hematology (*www.hematology.org/Patients/Your-Doctor.aspx*)

- Collect your medications, and know which ones might need a new prescription.
- Be ready to take notes about new information.

Medical History Outline

You know that people will ask you the same questions over and over again about your medical history. People with sickle cell disease can have complicated medical histories, so a smart healthcare provider will want to learn more about you before trying to start taking care of you. You might as well get ready by having the answers ready before your medical visit. Some families keep a "health passport." It might help a teen get familiar with his or her medical history to keep a notebook with key medical information.

- Do you know what type of sickle cell disease (hemoglobin SS, SC, S beta thal) you have?
- Do you know your baseline hemoglobin level?
- Do you know your baseline pulse ox level?
- Do you know all of your medication names and doses?
- Do you know all of your drug allergies?
- Do you know all of the surgeries that you have had?
- Do you know if you have received any blood transfusions?
- Do you know whether you developed antibodies because of past blood transfusions?
- Have you ever had a transfusion reaction?
- When you have sickle cell pain, how do you treat your pain? What activities ease your pain? What medications usually help you?
- Have you had any sickle cell problems like: stroke, acute chest syndrome, splenic sequestration, or sepsis?

One major problem in the United States is finding an adult doctor who will care for sickle cell adults. Start by looking for a hematologist with training in sickle cell. The next best physician would be an internist or family practitioner with an interest in sickle cell disease. Start at least a year before transfer is considered and ask your pediatric physician to help.

Children who have had strokes or have other disabilities may have special needs during transition. Guardianship, vocational rehabilitation, special funding, and other special provisions may be required. Social workers are an invaluable resource for helping with these needs.

7

Young Adulthood: Nineteen to Thirty-Five

MELISSA'S STORY

I was three years old when I was diagnosed with sickle cell disease. Living a few miles from the beach, it was just another day when my parents and I went to the ocean. It became a day unlike any other, though, when that night I was restless and ill, and nothing seemed to calm me.

In the morning my parents took me to our family doctor, and he arranged for me to have some tests, which over a series of weeks led to more tests. At one point, the doctors thought I had leukemia. My physician noticed my spleen was enlarged, and that, combined with the suggestion from my aunt, who was a nurse, to look into being tested for sickle cell, sparked my diagnosis. The test showed that this was just what I had.

Both of my parents had emigrated from Jamaica to the United States, and, although the disease is common in Jamaica, unfortunately neither of them had even heard of it. They didn't know that they each carried a gene for altered hemoglobin, which left them untouched but had a drastic effect on my own genetic make-up. The hemoglobin portion of my red blood cells (the part that carries oxygen to all of my body parts) was changed so that sometimes it caused my normal blood cells to sickle. My parents were told that I had the SC variant. Though my parents were from Jamaica, the same scenario happens every day here in the United States due to lack of information and lack of access to that information.

My parents were aware I had a disease, of course, but they tried not to emphasize that I might be different from anyone else. I also learned lessons the hard way, by sometimes denying my difference. For example, the kids in our fifth grade gym class were expected to run a mile to complete an end-of-the-year physical aptitude test. Instead of telling my instructor that I was tired, I pushed myself to exhaustion. I completed the run, but I missed the rest of the school year. The strains that triggered episodes weren't always physical. During my junior year in college, I was so stressed out about a test that I ended up in the ER. I was hospitalized only twice during my adolescence and young adult years. The fact is that the disease, in whatever form, does not affect everybody in the same way or with the same severity. Learning about the sickle cell trait was very important to me, because that trait had so much to do with who I am.

In Jamaica, about 10% of the population has the sickle cell trait, but, on other islands, the frequency varies from 7% in Barbados to as high as 13% to 14% in Dominica and St. Lucia. This compares to about 8% in the black American population, and frequencies of 20% to 30% in black populations of West Africa and of some populations in Saudi Arabia, India, Greece, and Italy. It's important to find out if you carry the sickle cell gene by getting a simple and painless blood test called hemoglobin electrophoresis. Getting tested is easy, and it can be arranged by your general practitioner or at your local sickle cell center or foundation. Soon, nearly everyone will be screened at birth.

When I was three, there wasn't much going on in sickle cell research or treatments. Twenty-odd years later, the outlook for someone like me who has the disease has improved tremendously. In the past, survival beyond the age of 30 was unlikely. Now it's common for many of us with the disease to live to old age.

There's still plenty of work to be done. In my community and many others, access to medical care can be difficult for a lot of people, but improvements are occurring as people learn more and more about how to find the medical help they need. I've made this my life's work. I received a master's degree in public health with health education—the focus of both my studies and my vision for the improved quality of life for those whom sickle cell disease affects. Where there's ignorance, there's myth, and myths surround sickle cell disease. Health education is about dispelling health myths. It's important to remember:

- Sickle cell disease is not contagious; it is a genetic disorder you have from birth.
- It is not cancer.

- The mind is not affected.
- It is not just a "black" disease but affects Hispanics and people of Asian and Mediterranean origin as well.
- It is not "bad blood" or a family curse.

Sickle cell is a disease that exists just as any other except in a way unlike any other. In its uniqueness, it offers challenges to both those who treat it and those who live with it. It is a disease that has molded my life and made me who I am and hope to be.

* * *

COMMON MANIFESTATIONS

Pain Episodes

Early adulthood is a period when many individuals with sickle cell have increased problems with their disease. Those with Hb SS and Sβ^0 thalassemia may have increased frequency and severity of pain episodes, increasing visits to the ER, and hospitalizations. Those with other forms may have the first onset of pain episodes and other complications. This occurs because of both rapid changes in biology and behaviors that create or increase problems with the disease. Both of these can be controlled, reducing problems during this period.

Most of our older adults who have lived through this period tell us that they had many more problems that started in the teens and lasted into the thirties. During this time, they just wanted to be normal, so they denied and ignored their disease and did everything their peers were doing. Many of these activities caused them to get sick. As they got older, they accepted their disease and took control of it. They learned to pace themselves, participate but stay within their limits, get adequate rest, and practice good health maintenance. Once they did this, their disease quieted down and they got on with their lives.

The biological factors that can be controlled are also important. Avoiding overexertion, staying hydrated, avoiding alcohol and street drugs, and following their treatment plan can reduce problems. Hydroxyurea should be considered by every young adult with sickle cell anemia and sickle thalassemia if they are not already on this preventive drug. If it is prescribed, it should be taken daily as directed by their doctor. Regular transfusions may be considered if the frequency of pain causes too much of a disruption to daily life.

You should learn how to manage your pain at home following your doctor's advice. Use a graded approach to your pain control based on the severity of the pain. Understand when you need to seek medical help for your pain episode, and use your pain medications responsibly by following instructions.

Gallstones

Gallstones are very common in individuals with sickle cell disease, occurring in up to 75% of individuals. This is a complication from an increase of bilirubin in the bile from the increased breakdown of the sickle cells. Most gallstones do not cause symptoms, but pain can occur from passing a stone, from a stone blocking the ducts draining to the liver or pancreas, or inflammation of the gallbladder (cholecystitis). Severe pain can be felt in the right upper or middle abdomen, between the shoulders blade or in the right shoulder. Eating may cause pain, and nausea and vomiting may occur.

Current recommendations are to watch gallstones if they are not causing symptoms. Surgical removal is required if they do cause symptoms, however. Minimally invasive laparoscopic surgery can usually be done with few side effects and rapid recovery.

Leg Ulcers

Leg ulcers cause chronic disability in 10%–15% of young adults with sickle cell anemia. Leg ulcers in those with sickle cell diseases start as a result of localized tissue death in the skin, which in turn is caused by clogging of small blood vessels with sickled red blood cells and blood clots.

Treatment includes the following:

- Medication. Many individuals with leg ulcers are deficient in zinc, and zinc is required for white blood cells to fight infection and for wound healing. Most individuals with leg ulcers should take supplemental zinc pills.
- Good nutrition.
- Prevention of swelling in the legs through elevation and by wearing supportive stockings is one of the most important treatment and prevention methods.
- Removal of dead tissue. This speeds healing and prevents infection by using hydrophilic dressings.
- Use of a zinc-impregnated bandage or Unna boot twice a week.
- Bioengineered temporary skin substitutes.

- Use of wet/dry dressings.
- Bed rest and leg elevation.
- Grafting. When leg ulcers cannot be healed by any other means, surgical skin grafting may need to be performed. This only works half of the time.
- Blood transfusion therapy.

It's always a good idea to exclude additional causes of ulcers, such as diabetes, peripheral arterial disease, and venous stasis, all of which have their own specific treatments.

The most important prevention is to avoid prolonged standing or sitting that causes the ankles to swell. Many ulcers may be prevented with good skin and foot care. If your skin tends to be dry and ashy, try using a good skin-lubricating lotion twice a day. Don't go around barefoot at home, in the yard, or at the beach. Splinters, bits of sharp metal, broken glass, or broken shells could be lurking there, ready to cut your skin and start the ulcer process. Avoid insect bites from mosquitoes, chiggers, and fleas. Always inspect your legs, ankles, and feet for areas that are painful and/or discolored when you get up in the morning and before you go to bed at night. Use a handheld mirror if necessary. Show any such areas to your doctor as soon as possible. Avoid buying unsuitable shoes simply because they look "hot"—they may rub on the ankle bone. Early care may help to prevent an ulcer from progressing and possibly becoming infected.

Osteonecrosis of the Hips and Shoulders

The round parts of the hip bone and shoulder bone each have small arteries supplying blood flow to keep the bone alive and healthy, but they can be blocked by sickled red blood cells. If this happens it can cause the round end of the bone to die. This condition, osteonecrosis (avascular necrosis), may be more common in Hb SC and Sβ^+ thalassemia type sickle cell disease but can occur in all forms of sickle cell disease.

In a patient with osteonecrosis, the affected area begins to collapse, making the round ball shape turn rough and jagged. This causes pain when walking or moving the leg at the hip joint and in the arm in the shoulder joint. Pain in the hip is felt in the groin, buttocks, and knee. The first line of treatment is to use daily arthritis medications that are safe (see the chronic pain treatment section), but the long-range objective is to prevent further joint destruction by taking weight off the hip through the use of a cane or crutch, and by limiting walking. The shoulder should be rested as much as possible. Physical rehabilitation has been shown to improve pain and functioning, and a physical therapist can help teach you how to exercise to maintain flexibility and strength without damaging the joint further. Vocational adjustments may be needed if one works on their feet all day, does heavy lifting, sits for long periods, or requires constant motion in the hip or joint.

If the pain level becomes too high and can't be controlled with medications or physical limits, a visit to the orthopedic surgeon for a consultation about a joint replacement should be scheduled. The surgeon may recommend an artificial hip or shoulder joint. Highly advanced new materials make these joints last much longer than previous models of artificial joints. Many doctors have changed their recommendations about joint replacement in young adults with sickle cell disease and suggest artificial joints at earlier ages than before. Ask your doctor to discuss how long an artificial joint might last in your situation, how much pain relief and function you might have, and how long you would need to devote to physical therapy rehabilitation exercise after a joint replacement. Older studies show that hip replacements do not last as long in young, active individuals and that many will have to be replaced because of infection, wear, and loosening, but more recent studies suggest much better outcomes.

The risks of joint replacement including postoperative complications, dislocation, joint infection, and joint failure are higher than in individuals without sickle cell disease. The surgeon should work with your sickle cell doctor to ensure the safest possible surgery, with a preoperative blood transfusion to raise your hemoglobin to 10, good hydration, and use of incentive spirometry (blow bottles) after surgery. After a hip joint replacement, rehabilitation exercise for several months with coaching by physical therapists will strengthen your muscles and make the joint stable again.

Eye Problems
Blocked blood flow in the small blood vessels in the back of the eye causes the eye to make new, weaker, blood vessels to bypass the blocked ones. These new blood vessels are thinner and tend to break open, causing bleeding into the clear eye fluid. This can also cause the retina, the seeing part of the eye, to detach. The result can be reduced vision or blindness.

Patients with Hb SC disease, and perhaps sickle beta plus thalassemia, may be at greater risk for these eye complications than those with sickle cell anemia. Yearly eye examinations by an eye doctor, with appropriate use of laser surgery, if necessary, may reduce the severity of these complications.

People with diabetes may develop a retinal disease that is quite similar to sickle cell retinopathy, or damage to the inner eye. Individuals with sickle cell disease and diabetes or hypertension may have higher risk of having retinopathy. Measures that have been successful in preventing the development and progression of diabetic retinopathy include reducing elevated blood pressure to not more than 120/80 and use of ACE inhibitors whether or not the blood pressure is high. We do not yet have any studies to prove whether these measures are effective for people with or at risk for sickle cell retinopathy. People with diabetic retinopathy are also told to avoid NSAIDs, constipation and straining, drink plenty of water, and eat plenty of fiber. There are no studies in sickle cell of these preventive measures, but it would seem logical that these measures would have the same effect for people with sickle cell disease.

REPRODUCTION AND PREGNANCY

Can people with sickle cell have children?
Yes, but planning is key. Sickle cell disease affects your ability to conceive a baby and carry it to full term, and there is increased risk of some complication. Sickle cell disease has lifelong implications that should be factored into the decision to have children. Raising children is hard work, requiring emotional and financial demands that may be much more challenging because of sickle cell disease.

Remember that sickle cell is an inherited disease. Your choice of a mate will directly affect the chances that your child will also have sickle cell disease. If your spouse has sickle trait, then there is a 50% chance that your child will have sickle cell disease. If you have sickle cell anemia and your spouse has normal hemoglobin A, then none of your children will have sickle cell disease, but all will be sickle carriers (have sickle trait). If your spouse is a carrier for beta thalassemia or some other hemoglobin that interacts with hemoglobin S, there is 50% chance that your child will have some form of sickle cell disease. (See Chapter 19 for more about genetics.)

Are men with sickle cell disease fertile?
Yes, but men with sickle cell disease may have a few issues that affect reproduction.

Priapism can leave scarring inside the penis can cause impotency—inability to have a normal erection of the penis. One of the reasons that an episode of priapism should be treated promptly is to relieve pain, but another reason is to avoid impotence. (See Chapter 6 for more about priapism.)

Sperm counts and sperm motility may not be normal in men with sickle cell disease. Sperm might also be affected by hydroxyurea, but it seems to recover when hydroxyurea is stopped. Many children have been conceived with men taking hydroxyurea, so it does not prevent pregnancy. However, the long-term effects of hydroxyurea on reproductive success in males are not known. Because there may be a risk of birth defects, men should not plan to father children while taking hydroxyurea. (See Chapter 13 for more about hydroxyurea.)

Are women with sickle cell disease fertile?
Yes, but women with sickle cell disease may be affected by several issues that affect reproduction.

Conception may be harder, and there is probably an increased chance of miscarriage in women with sickle cell disease. For some women, avascular necrosis of the hip joints makes intercourse painful and may prevent certain positions. Hydroxyurea should not be taken during pregnancy or while nursing because of concerns for the effects on the fetus. Hydroxyurea has been known to cause birth defects in laboratory animal tests, but after almost thirty years of study in humans, no increase in birth defects has been seen in women who became pregnant while taking hydroxyurea, though some women have had miscarriages. Women should discuss child-bearing plans with their doctor before becoming pregnant and should plan to stop hydroxyurea at least six to eight weeks before becoming pregnant. (See Chapter 13 for more about hydroxyurea.)

How is sickle cell disease affected by pregnancy?
Pregnancy causes demands on any woman's body. Good prenatal care is very important for every pregnant woman and for her baby. This is particularly crucial for a pregnant woman with sickle cell disease. The increased blood flow and nutrition for the baby in her womb can be a big strain for the heart and lungs of a woman with sickle cell disease. "Morning sickness" can cause anybody to become dehydrated, but dehydration comes even more quickly for a woman whose kidneys are affected by sickle cell disease. For

these reasons, pregnancy may be associated with worsening of sickle cell disease, including sickle cell vaso-occlusive pain. In our experience, most women have little change in frequency or severity of pain episodes, though many do have worse or more severe pain, and some actually have less.

Hemoglobin level falls during pregnancy in all women. In those with sickle cell, hemoglobin may fall to levels requiring transfusion. Studies also suggest that women who are transfused during pregnancy have fewer pain episodes. It is extremely important to take folic acid daily before and during pregnancy not only to prevent anemia but also to prevent serious birth defects in the baby. Most pregnant patients with sickle cell should be on prenatal vitamins and standard iron supplementation unless iron overload is present.

The placenta of a woman with sickle cell might be damaged by sickled blood cells, often causing the baby to be smaller than average. The risk of obstetric problems is especially high for mothers with sickle cell anemia (sickle cell disease SS). These problems may lead to the baby being born prematurely.

Management of pregnancy in the patient with a sickle cell syndrome requires carefully coordinated care by obstetricians and hematologists knowledgeable in the disease. Follow-up visits are usually scheduled every two weeks, with weekly visits when necessary for complications and during the last four to six weeks of the pregnancy.

Although complications have gone down over the last 20 years, there are still some increased risks for both mother and child. With careful management, there is no reason that women with sickle syndromes cannot have children.

Pregnancy in sickle cell disease should be a conscious decision and a planned event. All sickle cell patients should receive accurate information at puberty and periodically throughout their reproductive lives about the risks of pregnancy, genetic transmission of sickle syndromes, methods of contraception, prenatal diagnosis, prevention of sexually transmitted disease, and the increased responsibility of raising children.

Is the pregnancy and delivery the hardest part?
Perhaps not. Even with the deep joy of being a parent, any parent can tell you that raising a child is tremendously hard work. Caring for a newborn baby can mean sleeplessness for weeks, patiently figuring the needs of a

helpless creature who can't talk, and heavy lifting as the child grows. Caring for a preschooler means keeping watchful eyes on a fast-moving explorer who can't wait to taste, pull on, or climb everything within reach. Caring for a school-aged child means infinite patience with infinite questions: "Why?" Caring for a teenager means wisdom to know when to set limits consistently, when to show affection and encouragement, and when to simply listen and let go. And all of this requires the self-control to be a role model for the child watching how you do things.

These usual challenges of parenting can be very demanding for a parent living with sickle cell disease. It can be even more challenging if the child also has sickle cell disease. All mothers with sickle cell disease need an excellent support system to cope with properly raising a child. They should have a partner who can share the work-load and provide financial and emotional support throughout the process. Many parents will plan to live close to family and friends so that this support system can help with children when they themselves are sick or too tired.

Can I find out before birth if my baby has sickle cell?
Prenatal diagnosis can allow you to find out whether the fetus is affected by sickle cell disease. Genetic testing is done on a sample from the fetus. Probes or needles can be inserted into the placenta for chorionic villus sampling, which can be done early in pregnancy (between 9.5 and 12.5 weeks gestation).

This procedure may be somewhat risky for the fetus. The other prenatal diagnosis technique is amniocentesis (sampling the fluid sac around the baby), which can be done from about 14 weeks gestation to about 20 weeks gestation.

If sickle cell disease is present, you would have a head start on planning a treatment strategy for your child. You can save the cord blood from your child with a private cord blood bank, in preparation for possible gene therapy, though this is expensive. You will also have the option to terminate the pregnancy.

It is now also possible to ensure that a pregnancy will produce a baby free of sickle cell disease through in vitro fertilization (IVF), where the woman's egg is fertilized with sperm in the laboratory and put back into the woman's uterus. To avoid passing down sickle cell disease, only fertilized eggs without sickle cell disease are implanted.

PREVENTIVE MEASURES

In this age group, preventive measures for avoiding sickle cell issues include the strategies discussed previously under FARMS:

F—Fluids. Drink 8–10 glasses of water a day, and take 1 mg of folate every day. Folic acid may help produce more new red blood cells as well as help blood flow through smaller arteries.

A—Air—Avoid high altitudes, smoking, and asthma.

R—Rest when you need to, and don't overdo physical activity.

M—Medications like hydroxyurea may be the best preventive measure.

S—Situations to avoid: temperature extremes, alcohol, illegal drugs, and tobacco.

CLINICAL ISSUES

- Schedule clinic visits for a history, physical, and complete blood count (CBC) every two to six months. A reticulocyte count and urinalysis should also be done at each visit. Get blood chemistries, an eye exam, and a purified protein derivative (PPD) skin test for tuberculosis (TB) exposure once a year. Screen for gallstones and aseptic necrosis if symptoms occur.
- Keep immunizations up to date, and get an annual flu vaccination.
- Learn all about your sickle disease, pain management, prevention of complications, response to emergencies, and avoiding substance abuse.
- Learn the importance of hydration, diet, dental care, and knowing your limits.
- Ask your provider about disease variability, prognosis, and prospects for future therapy.
- Seek psychosocial support when needed.
- Learn how to do breast or testicle self-examination.

PSYCHOSOCIAL ISSUES

Young adulthood brings new challenges to everyone, and, as always, the challenges will be especially strong for people with sickle cell disease. New challenges faced by all young adults are establishing independence, choosing a career, developing new relationships, raising one's own family, and knowing how to accept and even seek the support of others. An additional challenge for individuals with sickle cell disease is taking charge of their disease by learning how to manage it so it has minimum impact on their quality of life—in other words, learning how to control the disease and not letting it control you.

Career Choices

Your first priority is to try and find a career that you enjoy and that supports your lifestyle. You will want to avoid jobs that could make your sickle cell disease worse. Many of our patients have their own small businesses or hold jobs where they can work from home to increase flexibility when dealing with disruption caused by the disease. However, many have very demanding occupations that tend to be outdoor jobs with exposure to temperature fluctuations or manual labor that can cause fatigue and increased sickling. Standing for long periods may cause pain in the hips and knees in areas with blocked blood flow and bone damage. It also may lead to leg ulcers or make them harder to cure. Find a career where you us your brain more than your body. We recommend jobs that are indoors, that are not manual, that have good health insurance benefits, and that are enjoyable. We encourage our patients to work hard in school and to go to college or vocational school studying subject they really enjoy. If you choose outdoor work, try to always dress appropriately for the weather, and, if possible, live in an area with mostly moderate year-round temperatures. Learn your limits and always try to work within those limits.

You should be honest with your employer about your sickle cell disease. It is good to work for an employer that understands sickle cell disease and knows that you may sometimes have to miss work because of pain events or other complications. Try and be a productive employee so they will feel comfortable accepting your absences. A letter from your doctor with information we have outlined in this book is a good start.

Family Issues

Many people with sickle cell disease choose to live near parents or brothers and sisters, who can help them when they need transportation, child care, help with household chores, and support when complications or severe pain episodes occur. Often, for the family, this is a continuation of a support system developed over a long period of time. However, it is also important that the adult becomes able to live an independent lifestyle and develop friends and other support networks.

Peer Support

A successful network for an individual with sickle cell disease will reach beyond the family to other individuals with disease, with whom one can offer and receive support and ideas, encourage and be encouraged, help raise community awareness, and advocate for excellent care in their local health care facilities. Communication within these groups can occur through newsletters, phone chains, e-mail, and the Internet. In addition, many of our patients in this age group have established networks on social media that provide support.

Formal support groups can be started with monthly meetings at a community-based sickle program, local home, a meeting room at the library, or a church. Alternatively, the hospital can help keep all informed about the latest news in the community.

8

Adulthood: Thirty-Six to Sixty-Five

INGRID'S STORY

My name is Ingrid Whittaker-Ware, Esq. I was born in 1962 to Raphael and Muriel Whittaker and was the fourth of five children. I was raised on the sunny island of Jamaica and immigrated to Atlanta, Georgia, in 1980.

I was diagnosed with sickle cell disease (SS) at eleven months old. Although I had signs of jaundice from birth, the doctors did not properly diagnose my disease until I was having an uncontrolled fever and crying more than usual for an eleven-month-old. I am the only one of my siblings to be born with the disease. Both of my parents have the sickle trait, as do one of my brothers and my little sister.

My parents taught me as a child the value and empowerment of knowledge and determination. Once, when I was having a pain episode, I cried and begged my parents to send me to school. I wanted this so badly that they let me go. That same day, during the lunch hour, I was hit in the head by a stray stone thrown by someone on the playground. The teachers wanted to call my parents right away, but I begged them not to, because I feared my parents would take me home and keep me out of school for several days until I was completely well. At that time, being in school helped to lift my spirits and take my mind off being more physically challenged than my peers. I was blessed to have had the expert and compassionate care of Drs. Elaine Reid and Graham Serjeant. To them both I owe a debt of gratitude for the care they provided me while I was growing up. Truly, I have been blessed from the time I was born. When I was diagnosed with sickle cell disease, the doctors did not expect me to live past my sixth birthday. In fact, at first I was diagnosed as having leukemia, and it was not until further testing that the doctors came up with the diagnosis of sickle cell disease.

Despite the gloomy predictions from the doctors, the good Lord is the author of my life and had other plans for me. So, He has always placed me in the care of the very best doctors in the area of sickle cell disease and research. Dr. Reid watched over me the only two times I was hospitalized as a child. The first of those two times I was not expected to live because of the seriousness of the infection. I was very young then and do not remember much about that hospitalization, but I do remember being placed in an oxygen tent and the grim expressions of the medical staff and my parents. Dr. Serjeant cared for me through adolescence into adulthood, and it was he who first taught me to protect my legs from insect bites and injuries in an effort to minimize leg ulcers.

I attended Spelman College, where I double-majored in political science and economics with a minor in international relations. I graduated *magna cum laude* in only three and a half years. Life at Spelman was fun. My professors inspired and challenged me to reach for the stars and further instilled in me the conviction that knowledge is power. For the most part, I stayed out of trouble with sickle cell disease at Spelman, although there were stressful times, what with the pressure of exams and the like. I viewed that type of stress as a positive challenge and managed never to have a serious pain episode for which I had to be hospitalized. I tried my best to take care of myself by hydrating myself constantly and following the healthy practices I learned early in life, which were reinforced by the staff at the Grady Sickle Cell Center.

I had several leg ulcers and one bout with what was suspected to be osteomyelitis while I was at Spelman. I remember my mother waking me up early one morning and asking why I was moaning. I told her that I was not moaning, but then immediately felt the pain in my ankle. This was the first time I was given a mild narcotic medication (Tylenol 3) to help control the pain. I could not do my usual activities that summer, which included working at a summer job. However, I refused to let the summer be an entire loss and decided to take a course in calligraphy. I am still able to write calligraphy today and sometimes get requests from family members to do a special piece for them. At Spelman, I also took time for piano lessons again, which I hadn't done since I was a child. Playing music, particularly the piano, often helped me relax and reduced my stress.

At Spelman, I won the prestigious Thomas Watson Fellowship. This fellowship gave me the chance to travel to Venezuela and extensively in Europe, in the quest of being a "better world citizen." On returning from my travels, in 1985, I enrolled in Columbia University School of Law in New York City. I graduated from Columbia and returned to Atlanta to work as an attorney for the federal government.

Whether I travel on business or for pleasure, I always take care to properly hydrate myself before, during, and after flying and have never encountered any major sickle cell-related problems due to air pressure. The air does sometimes become a little dry, but I counter that by breathing into a cup with a few drops of water or a few slices of lemon. A flight attendant taught me that trick while I was on one of the long flights from the United States to Venezuela when the dry air had become uncomfortable to breathe.

During my life's journey, as I have grown older, I have had many challenges. However, I have also had God's protection and His many blessings. Some of my challenges from sickle cell disease have included recurrent and painful leg ulcers and one aplastic crisis. The aplastic crisis racked my body with so much pain that I can only describe it as feeling like I had been hit by a runaway freight train. This aplastic episode was also accompanied by high fevers in excess of 105 degrees. I remember awaking from a feverish sleep to see my husband shivering with cold as he sat in the room with me. The doctors had drastically lowered the room temperature to try to bring my body temperature down. I also have frequent pain episodes (for which, thankfully, I usually do not have to be hospitalized), mild retinopathy, and require frequent blood transfusions (a fairly recent development). In addition, I had gallbladder disease and a heart attack before age forty. I have also had other illnesses that were not initially sickle cell-related but became so when sickle-related complications developed.

Despite the bleak outlook and shortened life expectancy predicted by doctors when I was first diagnosed with the disease, I am here to tell my story almost four decades later. I have also been blessed with a very supportive family, including a mother and father who had faith that their first daughter would survive and did everything in their power to ensure that I did. Their efforts included making sure they learned as much as they could about the disease and then passing that knowledge on to me so that I could, in turn, take care of myself. My parents maintained appropriate communications with my doctors while I was a child so that I could get proper and immediate treatment when necessary and ensured that I had a proper diet and nutrition. They also provided a comfortable, positive, and stable environment in which I could grow up. My three brothers, sister, and extended family and friends have also always been very supportive of me.

Today, I am married to Willie J. Ware Jr., my caring and supportive husband, who stands guard at my bedside each time I am ill. He hovers over me like a mother hen and gets on my case about taking care of myself as much as, or worse than, my mother does. I am also the proud mother of the cutest and most charming three-year-old toddler, William, who came into our family by adoption. I am fulfilled by having the joy and comfort of knowing that I am loved and cared about by not only my husband and son, but by my extended family and friends as well.

To my comrades in arms who live with the disease, I challenge you to:

- develop your spiritual life and ask for God's continued blessings, because—even when the doctors and everyone else give up hope—He is the only one who can bring you through the many trials that you face;
- adopt a positive attitude and know that with God's help you can do anything you put your mind to—so believe in yourself;
- believe that knowledge is indeed power—educate yourself as much as you can about your disease and your body, and take all the steps necessary to stay healthy and positive, including maintaining proper contacts with your healthcare providers and maintaining a healthy diet; and
- continue to have faith and hope that a cure to this disease will be found soon, and do whatever you can to contribute to that cause.

To caregivers, family, and friends, I say thank you—and continue to keep the faith. Keep yourself and your loved ones encouraged. The more you learn about the disease, the more you can help your loved ones and educate others in the fight against sickle cell disease. To healthcare professionals, again I say thank you. I also challenge you to continue to provide care in a compassionate fashion, treating your patients with the respect and dignity you would accord anyone who comes across your path. You never know—you could be entertaining a future lawyer, doctor, or influential person. Encourage your patients to live as full and productive a life as possible.

—*Written in 2001*

* * *

MICHELLE'S STORY

My name is Michelle Rodriguez. I was born in Brooklyn, N.Y., and I am 31 years old. I was born with sickle cell disease. My parents both had the sickle cell trait, though they didn't suffer from the disease. But they did have trouble with diabetes, heart disease, and high blood pressure that ran in both their families.

I don't remember much about how sickle cell struck me in early childhood, but when I was ten my mother told me that I had stayed in the hospital for two months after I was born while the doctors gave me blood transfusions and other kinds of IV treatment. As a young child I often had sickle cell attacks, and these attacks got worse as I got older. I did what I could with folic acid. I didn't do very well. My pain was often terrible and I grew weaker. My schooling was interrupted and almost ended by the disease. In junior high school, for instance, I missed two to three months of school each year. I tried hard to keep my life normal. I got through junior high by going to summer school for an extra semester. I was lucky to have a loving mother who taught me never to give up.

By the time I got to high school, the attacks got less frequent and less severe. I got through my freshman year very well. Then, in the beginning of my sophomore year, I got pregnant. As bad as this can be for any young girl, it was especially bad for me. During my pregnancy, I was in and out of the hospital all the time. I suffered severe joint pains from an infection the doctors couldn't pinpoint. When it came time for the delivery of the child, I was in crisis. I was suffering such severe joint pains and labor pains at the same time that I was never moved to the delivery room. Hooked to an IV and monitoring machines, torn by the double sets of pain that ran through me, I continued this terrible labor until, finally, the doctors had to deliver the baby by cesarian section.

I first saw my baby in the nursery, and I wanted to cry. She weighed only two pounds and five ounces, and it broke my heart to see this little infant already hooked to so many machines. I didn't think she'd live.

I'm happy to say that Dominique *did* live. Maybe she inherited that same courage my mother had taught me. I went on to graduate from high school. My sickle cell attacks became much rarer and less severe after my pregnancy.

But, shortly after I graduated, I had to have surgery, and when I was recovering the sickle cell attacks grew worse, and I was in and out of the hospital again. Much of my suffering is behind me, and finally I can say proudly that I have learned to live with sickle cell disease.

* * *

COMMON MANIFESTATIONS

Sickle Pain Crisis

Most patients experience fewer pain episodes as they get older. Our older patients report that this is because they get to know their disease and limits, and they work on making sure they do the things that prevent problems and keep themselves healthy. They take charge of their disease. Many individuals on hydroxyurea state that this helped them a lot, and that they have more problems when they forget to take it regularly.

Bone Pain

Most individuals without sickle cell disease develop increased aches and pains as they age. This is much more common and severe in older individuals with sickle cell disease. More prolonged and constant pain can be seen with repeated bone infarction, sickle arthritis, and avascular necrosis of the hip or shoulder. They may also develop osteoarthritis or rheumatoid arthritis, as do those without sickle cell disease.

With chronic pain, the safest medications for treating pain are non-steroidal anti-inflammatory drugs and acetaminophen. Opiates have limited value in treating chronic pain, and their chronic use and misuse can result in tolerance, physical dependency, and exacerbated pain in some. The use of hydroxyurea for bone pain can be discussed with your doctor.

There are numbers of physical and psychological techniques for pain management and control that can be learned, such as transcutaneous electrical nerve stimulation (TENS) units, relaxation techniques, and occupational and physical therapy approaches. These techniques may be useful in reducing pain and maintaining a functional lifestyle. The goal of therapy in chronic pain is not total relief from pain, but minimizing the severity, maximizing functioning, and maintaining the best quality life that is possible.

Kidney Problems

Sickle cell disease can alter kidney function in early childhood, and this progresses throughout life. With advancing age, damage that can lead to kidney failure becomes more common. The first sign of this damage is protein in the urine. All patients should be screened for protein in the urine annually, beginning at age six. If protein is found in the urine, the individual should be screened for high blood pressure and diabetes and be evaluated by a kidney specialist. High blood pressure and diabetes should be well controlled to prevent kidney and eye damage. Several blood pressure medications are being studied as ways of protecting the kidney from damage that leads to kidney failure. Anemia may get worse because the kidney does not produce enough of the hormone erythropoietin, which is needed to stimulate the production of red blood cells.

In the ten to fifteen percent of individuals who get kidney failure, dialysis is required to remove toxins and fluids normally filtered into the urine. Shots of synthetic forms of erythropoietin can be used to increase hemoglobin and prevent the need for transfusions. Individuals with sickle cell disease and kidney failure can benefit from kidney transplantation, and this treatment is available in several academic centers. Prevention of kidney disease is very important because treatments are difficult, and life is shortened once the kidneys fail.

Those with kidney problems should not take NSAIDs for pain or any other medication, including over-the-counter treatments, without consulting their doctor. Medications that normally are removed from the blood by the kidneys, including many opiate pain medications, must be carefully prescribed and monitored.

Lung Problems

Pneumonias, acute chest syndrome (caused by red cell sickling in lung blood vessels), and fat from bone marrow blockage are acute complications seen with increased frequency in patients with sickle syndromes. They are sometimes hard to tell apart because signs of chest pain, cough, fever, pulmonary infiltrates, and severe hypoxia are common to all. Treatment for acute lung problems involves careful monitoring of hemoglobin and blood gases, oxygen for hypoxia, IV hydration, pain treatment, and antibiotics. An exchange transfusion may be necessary in episodes with severe hypoxia, rapid progression, or diffuse pulmonary involvement.

Acute chest syndrome may be prevented by using incentive spirometry in all hospitalized patients. Good asthma care and yearly influenza vaccinations can also help to prevent acute chest syndrome and pneumonia.

Chronic restrictive lung disease from scarring is common in older individuals and can reduce oxygen in the blood. Smoking makes both reactive and restrictive lung disease worse, so it must be avoided. Hydroxyurea is proven to be useful in preventing repeated episodes. If the oxygen level is always low, then home oxygen may be prescribed to aid breathing.

Pulmonary Hypertension

Pulmonary hypertension, or increased blood pressure in the blood vessels carrying blood from the heart to the lungs, is a common complication in adults with sickle cell disease. If untreated, it can cause early death. The causes of pulmonary hypertension are multiple, including red blood cell breakdown (hemolysis), low levels of nitric oxide in circulation, chronic low oxygen levels, blood clots, and repeated blood-flow blockage with sickled red cells. It can be screened for with a Doppler echocardiogram. If this indicates a problem, then further testing, include a heart catheterization may be needed to determine the type and cause. Treatment includes hydroxyurea and treating for correctable causes. Exchange blood transfusions and specific treatment directed a primary pulmonary hypertension may be suggested.

Menopause

There are no reported research articles about menopause in individuals with sickle cell. At the same time, we have seen clinically that some women have more pain events and complications during this time period. Water loss during hot flashes requires additional water intake.

Bone health is a major concern, and annual bone density measurements are recommended. Although at any given age, black women have higher bone mass density than other groups, there are good reasons to believe that the bones of people with sickle cell disease are less dense and more fragile than those of others. Reasons for this include expanded bone marrow cavities to replace red blood cells; delayed puberty, with fewer total years of producing adult quantities of sex hormones; and decreased physical activity.

Vitamin D deficiency is almost universal in sickle cell anemia, and it should be monitored and replaced with calcium and vitamin D if it is low. Estrogen replacement may or may not be beneficial. The foundation of osteoporosis prevention and treatment is calcium. Before menopause, the recommended dosages are 1,200 mg of elemental calcium per day (in two or more divided doses taken with food) and 400 IU of vitamin D per day. After menopause, 1,500 mg of elemental calcium per day (in three divided doses taken with food) and 400-800 IU of vitamin D per day should be taken. An adequate diet should provide enough magnesium to help with calcium absorption, but if your diet is less than wonderful you should take a supplement of magnesium such as magnesium oxide. The use of bisphosphonates and other forms of osteoporosis treatment have not been studied. These can be considered but should be carefully monitored by a doctor knowledgeable in treatment of osteoporosis.

Hormone replacement therapy has not been studied in sickle cell disease, so the same cautions for all women such as risk of heart attack, stroke, breast cancer, and blood clots in the lungs and legs should be considered. Antidepressant drugs such as Cymbalta, Pristiq, Viibryd, Celexa, Zoloft or Prozac and the antiseizure drug gabapentin both do a nice job of reducing the frequency and severity of premenopausal and menopausal hot flashes and mood swings.

Vaginal lubricants such as KY Jelly may eliminate vaginal discomfort and dryness during sexual relations. Petroleum-based products like Vaseline should be avoided if a condom is used, as it breaks down latex and may result in leaks. Vaginal estrogen, also not studied in sickle cell disease, may be used at bedtime once or twice a week to help with vaginal thinning and loss of lubrication. It is available in cream form or easy-to-use tablets. Such treatment may also help with bladder control problems related to menopause. Vaginal estrogen used in this way is only minimally absorbed into the circulation and does not appear to be associated with increased risks.

PREVENTIVE MEASURES

In addition to normal FARMS prevention, men and women of this age should participate in cancer screening, including mammograms and Pap smears for women, and prostate screening in males based on current recommendations. Now that life expectancy for sickle cell patients is increasing significantly, older individuals with sickle cell need to undergo all of the healthcare screenings that are recommended for the general population of their age.

PSYCHOSOCIAL ISSUES

Most studies have shown that individuals with sickle cell disease do a very good job of coping with their disease and are well adjusted. Chronic pain, missing work, family pressures, depression, insomnia, and anxiety are the most common social issues in this age group. These can lead to further stress, anxiety, and depression. A professional counselor, social worker, clergy member, or psychiatrist can be a great benefit in managing these challenges. There are medications that help treat depression and chronic pain at the same time. A psychiatrist or your primary care doctor can prescribe these medications. (See Chapter 12 for more information.)

Peer Support
Meeting with other adults with sickle cell disease can help you relieve stress, share resources, and provide coping ideas for the pressures of life. The fellowship of other individuals with sickle cell can help build self-esteem and improve hope. Invite special speakers to address issues common to all. Get involved; volunteer to be a role model and mentor for younger sickle cell patients. Our transition program utilizes older individuals with the disease to interact with youth, giving their wisdom and answering questions. This is very beneficial for the youth, and our adults really find it rewarding to pass on their wisdom to the next generation.

Spiritual Issues
Patients with a solid spiritual foundation seem to do better physically and emotionally and are less depressive, experience less stress, and have a lesser fear of death. They also have a community of support when they are ill to help with family issues, transportation, meals, counseling, and encouragement. Consider becoming involved in your local place of worship.

9

Adults Over Sixty

A recent study from Jamaica reported on over 100 individuals with sickle cell anemia (Hb SS) who lived to more than sixty years of age. Forty were alive at the end of the study, and ages ranged into the 80s. Our experience and data from Georgia and California confirm that a small number of individuals with sickle cell anemia are indeed living this long, and that these older patients have a lifespan similar to the general population.

Individuals with sickle cell diseases now need to consider that they will have long lives and should think about issues like retirement and old age in addition to their disease. They also need to be followed and treated not only for sickle cell disease but for all of the diseases and disabilities that are commonly seen in the general population of this age.

SICKLE CELL DISEASE-SPECIFIC ISSUES

The frequency of pain crisis was reported to decrease in the older individuals followed in Jamaica; this was mirrored in our clinical experience in Atlanta. Pain episodes decrease, but arthritis and chronic bone pain tend to become more of an issue in these patients, and normal, age-related bone and joint problems may be increased.

Decrease in kidney function was also common in Jamaica. The hemoglobin levels seemed to fall with aging, and this may make weakness, fatigue, and shortness of breath a greater problem. Increased fetal hemoglobin levels due to genetics or hydroxyurea treatment were higher in these older individuals, so those taking hydroxyurea should continue to do so. Monitoring may need to be more careful because of decreases in kidney function and more sensitivity to side effects. Transfusions and administration of erythropoietin may be needed to support the hemoglobin level.

PREVENTIVE MEASURES

In this age group, the FARMS preventive measures are the same. Hydroxyurea should be continued with closer monitoring, and age-specific cancer screening, diabetes screening, and general health maintenance should be followed.

PSYCHOSOCIAL ISSUES AND SUPPORT

While adults who still work will continue to benefit from peer support and support on the job, those that retire will need to build on existing support from family, friends, and other social entities such as their churches. There is also an increase in losses of family and friends through deaths and diseases like Alzheimer's that can erode a support network. Older individuals with sickle cell disease have a wealth of information and experiences that they can share with others who have sickle cell and other serious illnesses that are common in this age group. Their practical and spiritual struggles make them experts on living with serious illness. There is much you can do for yourself and for others:

- Develop hobbies and interests to distract yourself from your disease.
- Get involved with fundraising or volunteering in the hospital that has served you.
- Become a mentor to a child, teen, or young adult with sickle cell disease or other illnesses. Your presence will be an inspiration to them. Help them work through the challenges you have already mastered.
- Be a camp counselor.
- Be a public speaker in your community.
- Get involved with politics to improve services for sickle cell patients.

This is a time to share your wisdom with the younger generation.

SPIRITUAL ISSUES

A 2016 study[1] demonstrated that out of 74,534 participants, frequent attendance (at least once per week) at religious services was associated with significantly lower risk of all-cause, cardiovascular, and cancer mortality. It is important to be involved with a faith community for support and well being.

---

[1] Li, et al. "Association of Religious Service Attendance With Mortality Among Women." *JAMA Internal Medicine* 176, no. 6 (2016): 777-785.

PART 3

•

LIVING WITH SICKLE CELL DISEASE

10

General Medical Care

You want to be sure that you and your loved ones get the best possible medical care. You can help do this by understanding not just your disease, but also the medical and non-medical teams that can help you, and the centers and agencies you can turn to for more information and support. You also need to know how best to finance the costs of health care. Finally, you need to know something about the tests the doctors use to monitor your condition and the means by which they provide new treatment when necessary. In this chapter, we'll introduce you to this information.

THE MEDICAL TEAM

Doctors

There is a wide variety of doctors who help care for sickle cell patients, each performing a different role:

Generalists: You will need a primary care physician who serves to coordinate your medical home. This may be a pediatrician, internal medicine doctor, or family physician. This doctor should be most familiar with all of your needs and problems and be the leader of the team of healthcare professionals providing your care. In some programs, the sickle cell doctor will serve in this role.

Hematologists are specially trained in blood problems, including sickle cell disease. These experts in sickle cell disease usually work in sickle cell centers in major metropolitan areas, but they may expand their availability through outreach clinics and telemedicine.

Ophthalmologists: You should have an annual eye examination with this doctor, who specializes in eye health. Your ophthalmologist, who should be familiar with sickle cell disease, will carefully evaluate the blood vessels in the back of the eyes to detect problems such as retinopathy.

Neurologists diagnose and treat strokes, headaches, TIAs, and other brain and nerve problems.

Pulmonologists treat asthma, chronic lung disease, pulmonary hypertension, and other lung problems.

Radiologists read X-rays and scans to help diagnose problems, and they often place special ports and IVs in order to draw blood and deliver medications into the veins.

Surgeons operate on gallbladders, spleens, and other organs when they develop conditions seen in sickle cell disease.

Urologists specialize in problems in the kidney and bladder that need surgery, and they also treat priapism.

Nephrologists treat kidney problems, including high blood pressure.

Obstetrician-gynecologists care for women's health needs, administer Pap smears, and manage pregnancy.

Cardiologists treat heart problems.

Orthopedic surgeons can operate on and replace hips and shoulders damaged by avascular necrosis.

Emergency medicine specialists are staff members in emergency rooms, skilled to handle emergency situations.

Anesthesia and pain specialists provide pain management and anesthesia for surgery.

Physician assistants (PAs) and nurse practitioners (NPs) are trained to do much of what doctors do and are supervised by doctors. PAs and NPs have special training in patient education and will spend time answering questions, doing medical checkups, seeing patients in the hospital, and coordinating care. By handling the routine care, PAs and NPs allow the sickle cell hematologist to see more patients, especially those with more critical needs.

Nurses

Nurses provide most of the "hands on" care in the clinic, hospital, and emergency room. They are teachers, medication providers, and care coordinators.

They also counsel patients and family members. Nurses are the caregivers in the hospital and are responsible for the 24-hour delivery of medications, monitoring your condition, and tracking your vital signs and fluids. Nurses can be specialists in areas such as pain management or critical care, or they can be generalists. Some nurses make home visits and can administer antibiotics and pain medication in the home.

Psychiatrists and Psychologists
Psychiatrists are medical doctors with special training in the use of medications to help depression, anxiety, and emotional disorders. Psychologists, who are not physicians, provide counseling, testing, and emotional support for the same issues. Both can be very important in your care because they can help you understand your feelings about your disease and your life, and they can teach you ways to cope with both the problems that stem from your disease and the stresses of daily life. It is important to have access to these members of the medical team when the need arises. Sickle cell is a lifelong condition that can cause emotional stresses that require professional help. Both psychiatrists and psychologists can teach patients how to use biofeedback, distraction, and relaxation techniques to help control pain. Psychologists can also help determine the cause of school problems through testing and counseling.

Social Workers
Social workers are trained to help others solve issues such as insurance coverage, job and school questions, housing problems, and medical disability. Social workers are experts in local support systems and funding sources. They do crisis counseling and help families get back on their feet after setbacks. Social workers are usually employed by hospitals, sickle cell centers, and health departments. The clinic or hospital social worker should be knowledgeable about the programs available in your state.

Chaplains
A healthy spiritual life is very helpful for maintaining hope and a positive outlook. Chaplains are clergy employed by hospitals and clinics to help meet the spiritual needs of patients. They are available for counseling about generalized fears, fear of death, depression, and emotional stress. Chaplains are also available to help resolve ethical questions that may arise in hospitals, clinics, and medical schools such as end-of-life issues, questions concerning clinical (human) research, and stem cell research. Many chaplains sit on

hospitals' human research committees, and many have training in psychology and social work, allowing them to serve patients more effectively.

Pain Management Specialists/Clinics
This diverse group of experts can be an important part of the care team for patients with sickle cell disease and with chronic pain. Chronic pain needs a different approach than acute pain episodes. Patients who have both acute and chronic pain often need management by these specialists.

This specialty is an outgrowth of anesthesia, and these experts include anesthesiologists, neurologists, sports medicine specialists, neurosurgeons, orthopedic surgeons, acupuncturists, chiropractors, acupressure therapists, biofeedback therapists, massage therapists, nutritionists, and herbalists. The best pain-management centers have staff members available from all or most of these disciplines. Unfortunately, the treatment that is selected for you may be as much a function of what your particular insurance covers as what is most medically appropriate for you.

Physical Therapists
Physical therapists are trained to help exercise and strengthen muscles and joints after surgery, injury, or bone infarction. They help train patients in *transcutaneous electrical nerve stimulation* (TENS) to block chronic pain. They can help instruct patients about how to keep damaged hips, shoulders, and other joints from getting worse.

Vocational Rehabilitation
These members of the healthcare team are experts in job training and retraining. They are aware of medical conditions like sickle cell and try to match patients with jobs that will not cause medical problems. If your job is causing you problems, this is the expert you want to see. In most states, having sickle cell disease qualifies you for vocational rehabilitation services, including retraining. Even better, see one of these experts before applying for a job or beginning job or career training. They are usually employed by state government or by rehabilitation programs. All states have vocational rehabilitation services. Information about each program can be found in a downloadable document at *www.fda.gov/downloads/AboutFDA/WorkingatFDA/UCM277757.pdf*.

Genetic Counselors
Genetic counselors are trained to interpret genetic lab tests and construct

special family trees called *pedigrees*. They can educate you about genetic diseases and counsel you on the risk of having a child with genetic diseases such as sickle cell, and they'll discuss all of the options that may be available to you. They are available at most university and other academic medical centers.

CLINICS

The best clinics for sickle cell patients have knowledgeable and compassionate staff members. You can get clinic recommendations from your local hematologist. You can also find out from other sickle cell patients where they get their care and if they are happy with the care. If you do not know any patients in your area, contact the nearest sickle cell association or sickle cell center for a recommendation. An updated list US of clinics, sickle cell associations, and centers by state is listed on the CDC's Sickle Cell Disease National Resource Directory at *www.cdc.gov/ncbddd/sicklecell/map/map-nationalresourcedirectory.html*.

If you have insurance with a managed-care organization (MCO, HMO or other), you may have an assigned caregiver and clinic. The clinician may be excellent, and MCOs are usually very good at preventive care. On the other hand, your clinician may have very little sickle cell experience. Ask the clinician for a referral to a sickle cell expert near your home. If the clinician can't direct you, ask the clinic administrators to direct you to the best sickle cell care available in your community. To thrive in a managed-care environment, it is necessary to be assertive—that is, politely insistent—if you sense that your care or your child's care is not going as it should. You will often have to be proactive if you or they feel you are not getting the treatment you need.

Sickle Cell Centers

Sickle cell centers offer the most comprehensive services and research programs, and the most diverse experience. Most of these centers are located in large cities. It may be worth your while to visit the nearest center regularly and to have a care plan developed for your local clinic, emergency room, and in-patient service. This allows your sickle cell care to be planned by individuals knowledgeable in the disease. The doctors, nurses, social workers, psychologists, nurses, genetic counselors, hematologists, educators and other clinicians in sickle cell centers often better know and understand the special needs of an individual with sickle cell disease. A primary care provider can meet many of your medical needs, but sickle cell patients often have special problems that make it worth the effort to see experts at one of these centers. Having such a plan in writing, signed by a physician, may also go a long way toward dispelling an unfortunate stereotype held by many emergency room staff that sickle cell patients, especially young black males, are often not truly having pain but are merely engaging in narcotic-seeking behavior.

Sickle cell centers are following the lead of the clinics in Atlanta, Georgia, and New York, New York. Many other cities have acute care facilities or day clinics to treat pain events outside of the usual emergency room. These facilities have a success rate of 80% or more in helping patients get better without having to be admitted to the hospital.

Emergency Rooms
Sickle cell patients usually rely on their local emergency room (ER) for pain management and emergent symptoms, but help yourself before you need to visit the ER. Have your regular healthcare provider write up and sign an emergency room plan with your medical history, physical findings, lab values, medications to use for pain, and your doctor's phone number. Have this plan placed in a notebook in your local emergency room, your electronic medical record, or in your hospital chart. Keep one copy to show the nurses and physicians in the emergency room when you do go, and always have this with you when you travel. You must be proactive when dealing with staff in the ER. For a particular geographic area, identify—*before* you need them—one or several nurse and physician champions for sickle cell patients—people who can make sure you get the proper treatment.

The NIH published evidence-based treatment recommendations in 2014 that are available to the doctor treating you at *www.nhlbi.nih.gov/health-pro/guidelines/sickle-cell-disease-guidelines*. Free, detailed sickle cell guidelines for healthcare providers are available around the clock, seven days a week, on the Sickle Cell Information website at *www.scinfo.org*.

Community-Based Sickle Cell Organizations
Many cities and communities have sickle cell foundations that provide sickle cell blood tests and community screening at health fairs and at high schools. These foundations provide support services that may include testing for sickle cell, genetic counseling, education, scholarships, summer camps, home visits, financial aid, transportation, and support groups. Services provided vary, so you need to contact your local program to find what is available. Most do not provide medical services, but a few founda-

tions have nurses and trained counselors on staff to provide limited medical care. Many of these groups know of healthcare providers in the community who have expertise and interest in sickle cell disease management.

The main national organization for the various community foundations is the Sickle Cell Disease Association of America (SCDAA). Its mission is "To advocate for and enhance our membership's ability to improve the quality of health, life and services for individuals, families and communities affected by sickle cell disease and related conditions, while promoting the search for a cure for all people in the world with sickle cell disease." They have developed a patient registry called "Get Connected." The SCDAA publishes and distributes, to parents and teachers, educational materials for living and coping with sickle cell disease. There are links to Get Connected and many other resources.

The contact information for SCDAA is listed in the resources section of this book. Their website, *www.sicklecelldisease.org*, has a listing by state of all of their member organizations and their contact information. The local office of SCDAA is a valuable resource for help and support. You may also wish to volunteer at the local office and become a resource yourself.

COST OF CARE

The least expensive treatment is preventive care—regular checkups with your sickle cell provider. This is about $300 per visit. A sickle cell patient's biggest cost is the hospital charge for in-patient stays. The average hospital stay for a sickle cell patient is five days, at a cost of $20,500. Preventive measures that reduce the need to stay in the hospital will reduce costs dramatically. The cost will vary city to city and hospital to hospital. Visits to the local emergency room account for the next largest expense, which varies depending on your location. In 1,400 sickle cell patients followed at the Georgia Comprehensive Sickle Cell Center at Grady Hospital in Atlanta, Georgia, the average number of emergency visits per year is three, and the need for admission has decreased to an average of one every two years.

Medications such as penicillin and folate are inexpensive. The preventive medication hydroxyurea costs under $1 a pill, and one or more pills must be taken daily. Many drug companies have patient support programs that help you get the medication if you can't afford it. These programs usually require paperwork filled out by your doctor.

Cost for lab work and X-rays can add to the bill. The most expensive test is the MRI, which runs about $1,500.

Bone marrow-stem cell transplant can cost nearly $300,000. Insurance companies must approve this procedure ahead of time.

What if I Don't Have Insurance or Money to Pay for Care?
The Patient Protection and Affordable Care Act (PPACA), better known as "Obamacare" or the Affordable Care Act (ACA), is a law passed by the federal government to improve the state of health insurance in the US. The goal of the ACA is to make healthcare coverage better, cheaper, and more accessible to all Americans, which in turn would cut the cost of healthcare for individuals as well as the government. The law also requires insurance companies to provide coverage to everyone who applies for it, even if they have a pre-existing condition such as sickle cell disease. Visit *www.healthcare.gov* for more information and to start your registration process.

Programs like Medicaid, available to people who meet financial eligibility requirements in all states and territories of the United States, can pay for practically all of your or your child's medical care if you qualify.

The specific requirements an individual or a family must meet to qualify for Medicaid vary from state to state. The best source of information on your state's requirements is a social worker or the local Medicaid office.

Medicaid's stated policy now is to place most subscribers into Medicaid-HMOs, but patients or their parents can apply for exemptions, which are usually granted in the case of serious, chronic illnesses like sickle cell disease. More information about Medicaid eligibility and services can be found at *www.cms.hhs.gov/medicaid/consumer.asp*.

The State Children's Health Insurance Program (SCHIP) is a program supported by both the federal and state governments, providing health coverage to uninsured children whose families earn too much to qualify for Medicaid but too little to afford private coverage. All states provide free immunizations and well-child care at no cost. For details see *www.benefits.gov/benefits/benefit-details/607*.

What If I Have Insurance but Find My Options Confusing?
If your employer offers healthcare insurance, arrange to talk with someone in your personnel or benefits office who can guide you to the best available options for your child and family.

If you work for a small business and no such counseling is available, seek the advice of a social worker. Many hospitals, clinics, YMCAs/YWCAs, houses of worship, and community groups offer the services of a qualified social worker for free or for a nominal charge.

If no such community-based resource exists in your area, consider hiring an independent social worker in private practice. You can find social workers and their contact information online at *www.helpstartshere.org/find-a-social-worker*. Friends, neighbors, doctors, nurses, and clergy are good people to ask for referrals to social workers. Usually one or two visits with a private social worker are affordable and well worth the investment.

Knowing the Details of Your Health Plan

Whatever your health plan, it pays to read it carefully and to know its regulations. If you are denied authorization for a test or treatment that your child's doctor has ordered, *be politely assertive*. You don't have to accept a "no" from the lowest-ranking person on the authority ladder. If you're not satisfied with the answer you get, ask to speak to the next person up the ladder, and so on. *Polite persistence often carries the day*. This is especially true if you belong to a managed care plan.

Working with Health Maintenance Organizations (HMOs)

HMOs assign patients to a primary care provider (PCP). This provider may be a family practitioner, a pediatrician, an internist, a gynecologist, a geriatrician (a specialist in the care of older adults), a physician's assistant, or a nurse practitioner.

The PCP is in charge of your overall care and acts as a medical home for your care. They also often serve as a *gatekeeper*—that is, if you are the parent of a child with sickle cell disease, the PCP determines what tests your child will have, what treatment will be recommended, and whether a specialist should be consulted.

The guiding rule of an HMO is to maximize preventive care to keep you healthy and to keep its costs low. This means that it tends to do certain things well and other things not as well. HMOs usually do a good job of preventive care because preventing complications saves them money. That means they are good at making sure your child gets the proper immunizations, which is key to reducing the frequency and severity of crises. They also, usually, do a fine job of nutritional counseling, because good diet is important in making sure that your child grows as big and strong as the disease allows, and that the child's anemia is held in check.

But you may start to run into resistance with your HMO when it comes to treatments. Your PCP may choose a less expensive treatment, or the most effective treatment based on evidence. This will limit your access to new and not well established treatments that you hear about on TV.

The PCP may limit your child's access to a blood specialist (hematologist)—who is an expert in treating sickle cell disease—outside of the HMO, because such outside consultations cost the HMO more money. In other cases, the PCP may prefer to put most of your child's care in the hands of a specialist rather than tie up his own limited office time in the care of a complicated case.

Some HMOs might not pay for more aggressive treatments for sickle cell disease, like bone marrow transplantation. They argue that such programs are experimental, even though their usefulness in selected patients has been well established.

If you are denied a treatment or service that you think you should have, remember that HMOs have an appeals process. This process will often result in approval of the treatment if it is proven to be cost effective; that is, it works and reduces the overall cost of your treatment.

Working with Preferred Provider Organizations (PPOs)
A PPO, or preferred provider organization, is another kind of managed care plan. In this type of plan, you should have a generalist who serves as a medical home, but you may be able to see any specialist who participates in the plan *without* referral from a PCP.

Some PPOs will even pay a portion of the fees for visits to doctors outside their network, although you will be responsible for a larger portion of the fee than if you saw a doctor within the network.

Lately, PPOs have introduced reforms that allow tests—for example, certain imaging procedures—that they previously did not support. PPOs often require prior approval for procedures, and, while their prior approval staff is usually pretty reasonable, the extra time involved may stop some doctors from ordering tests that require such approval.

Working with Traditional Fee-for-Service Plans
The traditional fee-for-service plan is the third major type of health plan. In

this type of plan, which is becoming ever-rarer and more expensive, you can see any doctor you want. After an annual deductible (which varies from one plan to another) has been met, the plan will pay the doctor 70%–85% of the *approved amount* for the doctor's services. The approved amount is usually significantly less than the doctor's standard fees.

If your child's doctor accepts assignment, you usually will only be responsible for the portion of the approved amount not paid by the plan. If your child's doctor does not accept assignment, you will be expected to pay the doctor directly for your child's care. The plan will then reimburse you the usual percentage of the approved amount.

Working with Medicare
Your child may be able to get Medicare coverage if he or she is awarded Social Security disability. For a child to qualify, he or she must have worked on a job that withheld Social Security taxes. To qualify, your child must stop working because of his or her medical condition. Information about Medicare is available at *www.medicare.gov*.

Working with Disability/SSI
Another Social Security program for the disabled is SSI, or Supplemental Security Income. To be awarded SSI, a person has to fulfill the same requirements as for Social Security disability, except that the applicant does not need to have been previously employed. The financial award is usually less than what one receives with a disability award. This program does not lead to Medicare coverage. Sickle cell complications may not allow you to do any substantial work. You can find information and apply online at *www.ssa.gov*.

Falling Through the Cracks
Some people just don't qualify for any federal assistance program. Individual states, however, have begun to respond to this vacuum in federal programs. For instance, states offer a low-cost health insurance program for children, usually called Children's Health Insurance Program (CHIP), which covers many of a child's basic healthcare needs. A social worker can tell you the particulars of your state's program.

Many sickle cell clinics will try to provide care to you or your child at reduced fees or at no charge, if you are unable to pay. Many public and private voluntary hospitals will provide medical care, including high-caliber specialty care, on a sliding fee scale. Establish residence in a county with a county-supported public hospital. Check out the public health clinics in your city or county for preventive care and immunizations. A list of public "safety net" hospitals that provide care for low-income, uninsured patients is available at *www.essentialhospitals.org*. Again, a social worker can advise you.

COMMON LABORATORY (LAB) TESTS
Complete Blood Count (CBC) and Reticulocyte Count (Retic Count)
The most common blood test is the CBC. This is actually several blood tests combined into one. It lets your healthcare provider know how you are doing by the numbers of cells in the blood. Some tests count the number of red blood cells, white blood cells, and platelets. Others measure the *hematocrit*, which is the percentage volume of red blood cells over the total volume of blood. There is also a measure called the mean corpuscular volume (MCV), which checks the average size of the red blood cells. If the red cells are larger than normal, it might mean you are low in folate or vitamin B12, or this can simply be a side effect of being on hydroxyurea. If the red cells are smaller than normal, it may mean that you are low in iron, have a thalassemia, or have lead poisoning. The hemoglobin value is also reported.

Your healthcare provider closely monitors these blood values. Each person has his or her own usual values. In a person with sickle cell disease, a change in the blood values, either higher or lower, can be a sign of serious complications.

The best way to see if the bone marrow is making new red blood cells fast enough is a test called the reticulocytes count. The white blood cell count is important to watch, because it often rises when the body is under attack from viruses or bacteria. Platelet count is higher than normal in sickle cell anemia patients, and it can be lower than normal with some sickle cell disease complications or if the spleen is too big.

Blood Chemistry Values
A blood chemistry value that is important to know about in sickle cell disease is the LDH, or *lactate dehydrogenase*, an enzyme found inside red blood cells. In sickle cell patients, this value is usually higher than normal because of the constant splitting of sickled red blood cells in 14 days (hemolysis), rather than the normal 120 days. Another chemical released from the breakup of red blood cells is indirect *bilirubin*, a by-product of hemoglobin recycling. When bilirubin levels go above 2.0 mg/dL, the white part of the

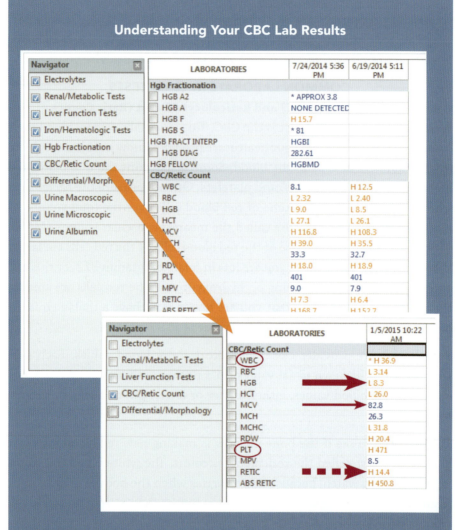

Understanding Your CBC Lab Results

What are the key parts of the blood counts (CBC and reticulocyte count) that I need to understand when reviewing my lab results?

- The thickest arrow is on **hemoglobin (Hgb or Hb)**. Lower numbers mean more severe anemia.

- The dotted arrow shows the **reticulocyte** percentage. Higher numbers mean more red blood cells are newly produced.

→ The thin arrow is on **Mean Cell Volume (MCV)**. Higher numbers mean bigger red blood cells. Higher MCV is one of the helpful effects of hydroxyurea treatment.

WBC is white blood cell count. Higher numbers mean inflammation or infection, or other stress to the body.

Plt is platelet count. The platelet count can change in many sickle cell conditions.

The lab sheet lists so many results as abnormal. How do I interpret my own CBC and reticulocyte results?

Having sickle cell disease makes many of your CBC results fall outside the ranges for people without any blood disorder. But looking over your CBC and reticulocyte results with your doctor can show you that many results always are the same when you are doing well. These are your own "baseline" CBC results.

Do the CBC and reticulocyte results measure pain?

It is important to know that pain cannot be measured with the CBC, the reticulocyte count, or with any other blood test available (as of 2015). You can still have sickle cell pain or other medical problems while your CBC and reticulocyte counts are "normal" for you, meaning they are at your baseline.

What if the CBC and reticulocyte results are not at my baseline?

Interpreting why CBC or reticulocyte results are not at baseline in people with sickle cell can be very complicated. Not every doctor learns these skills. That is one of the biggest reasons why you should see a hematologist, or another doctor with a lot of experience treating sickle cell disease. Your hematologist can advise you on what to do and what treatment options are available to get your CBC and reticulocyte results back to your baseline.

eyes becomes yellow. This is not harmful, and it comes and goes with the amount of red blood cells breaking apart. Bilirubin also goes up when the liver is not working well or gallstones are causing problems.

The alanine transaminase (ALT), aspartate aminotransferase (AST), albumin, and alkaline phosphatase (ALP) values also can indicate how the liver is doing. When the liver becomes irritated by infection or gallstones, these values rise. Sickle cells getting stuck in the liver can also cause these values to be high.

The blood urea nitrogen (BUN) and creatinine values indicate how the kidneys are doing. They go up when the kidneys are less efficiently filtering toxins from the blood. There are many other chemistry tests that are measured to diagnosis and follow complications.

Urinalysis and Urine Protein
A urinalysis consists of multiple tests on a sample of urine to check how the kidneys are working and to see if there is blood or infection in the kidneys or bladder. Too much protein released by the kidneys into the urine is one of the first signs that the kidneys have been damaged by sickled red cells. Research is ongoing to find ways to prevent this damage using special blood pressure medications and other drugs. Sickle cell patients should be screened at least every year for protein in the urine.

Ferritin
Ferritin is the best simple blood test to measure the level of iron in the body. As patients have repeated blood transfusions, iron builds up in the body. Ferritin levels indicate how much iron has built up. Iron deposits in many organs, like the liver and heart, causing damage. In order to get rid of excess iron, a medication called a chelator must be taken. Individuals with sickle cell may also be low in iron, and the ferritin is an accurate test of whether there is enough iron in the body to make new red blood cells.

Hemoglobin Electrophoresis
Hemoglobin electrophoresis is the blood test that determines the types of hemoglobin that are in the red blood cells. This and other methods of hemoglobin diagnosis are discussed in the diagnosis detection chapter. Clinicians will do repeated checks of the hemoglobin S level with this test, when a patient is on monthly blood transfusion therapy, to make sure the treatment goals are being reached.

Looking for Infection

Fever is the most important sign of infection. The white blood count will often be checked when you are being treated because it can also indicate that infection is present. When clinicians suspect an infection, they may order cultures of the urine, blood, throat, sputum, joint fluid, or other body fluids to see if bacteria are growing and, if so, to identify them. Cultures usually take 24 to 48 hours to reveal if bacteria are present. Because waiting for the results could be deadly, an antibiotic is commonly given to protect the patient while waiting for the test results. New tests are also being developed that can diagnose infections faster by looking for DNA or proteins from the bacteria.

Other tests for infection include blood tests that detect the presence of viruses like influenza, human immunodeficiency virus (HIV), viral hepatitis, mononucleosis, and cytomegalovirus (CMV).

Chest and dental X-rays, bone and gallium scans, and tagged white blood cell scans may also identify where infections are in the body.

COMMON TREATMENTS AND PROCEDURES

Intravenous (IV) Fluids

Sickle cell pain and complications can be made worse by a lack of water inside the red cells. A quick way to put the water back into the red cells is by drinking water or receiving IV fluids. A small plastic tube is placed in a vein, and water with glucose (sugar) and small amounts of sodium (salt) is allowed to drip into the blood stream. Drinking water can have the same re-hydrating effect, but it is difficult to drink enough water when pain is present or medications are causing nausea. IVs are also used to put other medications directly into the blood.

Transfusion Therapy

Blood transfusion is a very important treatment in sickle cell complications. It is often necessary when the number of red blood cells becomes too low; to treat or prevent a stroke; to treat acute chest syndrome, splenic sequestration, and persistent priapism; and to reduce the number of pain episodes if they are very frequent. Transfusions are given before surgery to prevent complications. In a *simple transfusion*, a bag of donor red blood cells is dripped into vein by an IV over a few hours. An *exchange transfusion* involves removing sickled blood cells from the person while transfusing in the donor red cells. This may be necessary in emergency situations or when

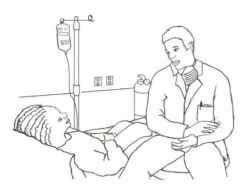

the sickled red cell count is too high in order to lower the percentage of red cells containing sickle hemoglobin. Exchange transfusion is also done monthly to prevent iron overload in individuals receiving chronic transfusions.

Transfusions are frequently needed for sickle cell complications. They can prevent complications like stroke and pain episodes and can be lifesaving in acute chest, splenic sequestration, and other severe complications. Although generally safe, there are several important complications that may occur with transfusion. The more common ones include too much blood volume (overload), alloimmunization (explained below), and iron overload. Exposure to infections is rare with the extensive testing that is now done on blood, but this is still feared by many. Fluid overload is usually caused by doing the transfusion too quickly without allowing the body enough time to adjust to the extra red cells and fluid. Increasing the hemoglobin level too high also can cause a stroke or a pain episode from the blood sludging, or becoming thick and slow-flowing).

Alloimmunization is a common problem occurring in about one quarter of transfused sickle patients. The patient's immune system begins to react to the donor blood cells and attacks them. This causes a delayed transfusion reaction in which the transfused cells are destroyed. It can also cause the body to develop antibodies—called autoantibodies—that destroy the individual's own red blood cells, making their hemoglobin level fall lower. Both allo- and autoantibodies make it difficult to find a blood donor that is a match. Individuals with sickle cell disease should be screened for antibodies and the antigens (proteins) on their red blood cells determined before they are first transfused to prevent transfusion reactions in the future. They should be screened for new antibodies before every transfusion. You can help prevent alloimmunization and delayed transfusion reactions by giving your healthcare providers a record of previous transfusions, reactions, and alloantibodies.

Alloimmunized individuals should wear an identification bracelet that provides alloantibody information, a record of the best blood for the patient based on the antigens on his or her red blood cells, and a number to call to obtain the patient's transfusion history. Screening for alloantibodies six to eight weeks after transfusion, although not usually done, will document new antibodies. These may disappear if there is a prolonged period without transfusion, but they can still cause delayed transfusion reactions if further transfusions are required. The likelihood of causing antibodies to develop can be reduced by using donors of the same ethnic background as the patient. Limiting the number of units transfused is also important.

Iron overload occurs in all individuals who receive many transfusions. The hemoglobin in the transfused red cells releases iron when the cells are broken down and the body has no way of getting rid of the iron. Iron overload can also be prevented by limiting the amount of red blood cells transfused. Exchange transfusion, in which sickled blood is removed as new donor blood is transfused in, is another method of limiting iron overload. There are also a number of iron chelators that can be given to treat iron overload.

Infection is now rare because blood that is to be transfused is extensively screened for infections such as hepatitis, HIV, West Nile virus, and others. Donors are also carefully screened for increased risk of these infections, and only volunteer donors are used. Individuals requiring transfusion should be immunized for hepatitis and should be tested for hepatitis (especially hepatitis C) or HIV on request. It is actually much more common to acquire these infections by way of unprotected sexual contact (especially hepatitis B and HIV), by contaminated food or water (especially hepatitis A or B), or by the use of street drugs through the IV, skin popping, or snorting routes, where the "works" (needles or straws) are either shared or not adequately sterilized.

Records of all transfusions, reactions, and alloantibodies are extremely important for all patients and parents to carry at all times. These should be updated after every transfusion recording the amount given, reactions, and new antibodies detected. These should be presented to any new physician and to those giving transfusions. A running total of units transfused will help track the iron put into your body.

Chronic Blood Transfusion

Monthly transfusions of normal red blood cells can greatly reduce the risks of major sickle cell complications such as stroke and acute chest syndrome. Chronic transfusion may help individuals with frequent pain episodes and those with pulmonary hypertension. They may also become necessary if kidney or heart failure develops. Chronic transfusion often causes iron overload, which can be reduced with daily use of iron chelation medicines. If iron overload is not managed properly, it can cause liver, heart, and hormonal problems.

Exchange transfusion, or *erythrocytapheresis*, is a special type of chronic blood transfusion. Blood is taken away from the body while new red blood cells are transfused. The advantages of exchange transfusion are greater replacement of normal blood cells for sickle red blood cells and less iron overload. Disadvantages of exchange transfusion include a greater exposure to red blood cell antigens and infection, a much higher cost, and the fact that it requires many more units of blood, placing a greater demand on the blood bank.

Chelation Therapy for Iron Overload
The human body holds on to iron very tightly. Iron overload can occur in people with sickle cell syndromes who have had many red cell transfusions. The body's iron stores become full after receiving approximately 20–30 units of blood by transfusions. More iron accumulation beyond this point may lead to problems in the liver, heart, and endocrine organs. In sickle cell disease, the liver seems to be the organ most affected. The heart may also be affected by severe iron overload leading to heart failure and rhythm problems. All endocrine glands may be affected, but the most commonly affected are the pancreas, leading to diabetes mellitus, and the anterior pituitary. Pituitary problems, in turn, may cause short stature by depriving children of growth hormone; sexual, menstrual, or reproductive problems by depriving people of sex hormones; low cortisol; low thyroid hormone; and failure to produce milk for your baby after giving birth.

While the blood test that determines your serum ferritin level is the easiest and most frequently used measure of total body iron, the level of hepatic iron concentration (HIC) is considered to be the most accurate measure. This test involves analyzing a sample of the liver (liver biopsy) and is done by a specialist. New types of magnetic resonance imaging (MRI) can accurately estimate iron stored in the heart muscle and in the liver.

Deferoxamine mesylate (desferrioxamine, Desferal, DF) is an injectable iron chelator (iron remover). Iron bound to DF is excreted in the urine and turns the urine pink. DF is not well taken through the stomach and is rapidly cleared from the blood, so it is only effective for chronic chelation therapy when given through a needle for many hours a day every day. DF has been in regular use for treatment of transfusional iron overload since the mid-1970s. It is most frequently given using a small pump to infuse the drug under the skin over 8–12 hours at least five nights a week. Deferoxamine treatment can be difficult for patients and their families because of needles, pumps, long treatment times, and the hassle factor.

Initiation of deferoxamine therapy should be considered if, after 20–25 transfusions, any of the following occur:

- Transferrin saturation (Fe/TIBC ratio) is greater than 80%.
- Ferritin level is 2,000 ng/mL (nanograms per milliliter) or higher.
- Hepatic iron concentration is greater than 3 mg/g of dry weight.

Management of iron overload should involve a healthcare provider who is an expert in its treatment. Before starting DF therapy, tests of hearing, vision, heart function, liver function, kidney function, and growth and development are recommended. Annual reassessment of these parameters, as well as calcium metabolism and endocrine function, is suggested.

Besides deferoxamine, there are two other medication-based options for iron chelation. The first oral iron chelator, deferiprone, was developed 20 years ago as a three-times-a-day treatment. It is less effective than deferoxamine, but it is easier to use. The side effects include joint problems and a low white blood cell count. Deferasirox (Exjade), a once-daily oral iron chelator that is mixed in liquid and swallowed, was approved by the US Food and Drug Administration in 2005. A new formulation of deferasirox (Jadenu) is a pill taken once a day that was approved by the FDA in 2015. According to the drug's safety information, deferasirox treats chronic iron overload due to blood transfusions in patients who are at least two years old. Potential risks of deferasirox include kidney and liver problems as well as bleeding in the stomach or intestines.

Another approach to iron overload that may be possible is to slowly switch from chronic transfusion to treatment with hydroxyurea. If the patient's hemoglobin level goes high enough, blood can be removed on a regular basis, reducing the amount of iron in the body. This has been shown to be effective in selected individuals who had been transfused chronically because of a high risk of stroke.

Ultrasound

Ultrasound painlessly uses sound waves to bounce back images of body organs. It can detect gallstones, spleen size, kidney size, and if a baby is doing well in the mother's womb.

Echocardiogram

This is a special type of ultrasound that examines the heart. It can measure how the valves in the heart are working, the size and thickness of the chambers of the heart, and how well the heart muscle is squeezing. An echocardiogram can also detect backwards blood flow through one of the valves of the right heart (tricuspid valve regurgitation velocity), an important marker of possible abnormally high blood pressure in the lungs (pulmonary hypertension). The silent problem of pulmonary hypertension is important to detect by screening echocardiogram.

Exercise Test and Six-Minute-Walk Test

Exercise tests can measure how well your heart and lungs are functioning. The six-minute walk test means walking back and forth in a 100-foot hallway with a hard, flat surface as quickly as you can. A technician will use a stopwatch to say when six minutes are up but is not allowed to give you coaching or encouragement. A bicycle exercise test involves pedaling a stationary bike while connected to probes that measure heart rate and oxygen level and run an electrocardiogram. A treadmill exercise test is much like a bicycle exercise test, but it involves walking or running on a treadmill that becomes a ramp, also while connected to probes. These tests can be done safely with standardized techniques.

Pulmonary Function Tests

Pulmonary function tests show how much air the lungs are moving in and out. They can indicate if a person has asthma, chronic obstructive lung disease, or reduction in lung volumes from scarring. A test, D_{LCO} (diffusing capacity of the lung for carbon monoxide), may be done to estimate how well oxygen is getting from the lungs to the blood. In sickle cell disease, it's important that the lungs work well, because anything that interferes with oxygen getting to the red blood cells will increase the sickling inside the body.

Eye Examinations

Sickle cell disease, especially type SC and sickle β^+ thalassemia, can cause damage to the blood vessels in the back of the eye. This can lead to bleeding and retinal detachment that causes loss of vision. The signs of early blood vessel damage can be seen by eye doctors, and treatment using lasers can prevent future damage. *We recommend that all sickle cell patients have a complete eye examination by an ophthalmologist, who can look in detail at the retina, once a year to check for this early damage.*

Hearing Tests
Sickle cell disease can cause damage to the nerves involved in hearing. Hearing tests are important to detect hearing loss and prevent school, work, family, and relationship problems. Annual hearing tests are recommended if a patient is receiving iron chelation therapy.

Transcranial Doppler (TCD)
Transcranial Doppler (TCD) is another painless ultrasound test that measures the speed and turbulence of blood flowing through the large blood vessels supplying the brain. When a blood vessel is about to close over because of sickle cell damage, it works a little like blocking the end of a running hose with your finger—the water comes out faster, with increased sound. The TCD is the best way to predict which children are at risk for having their first stroke. Such cases can be treated with blood transfusion therapy to prevent strokes before the first one happens.

Computerized Tomography (CT) and Magnetic Resonance Imaging (MRI) Scans
A computerized tomography (CT) scan is a special X-ray that allows a cross-sectional view of the organs in the body. CT can detect the presence of stroke, blood, tumors, growths, swelling, and blockages within the body. Special CT scans of the chest are used to show blood clots in the arteries of the lungs.

Magnetic resonance imaging (MRI) uses a large, powerful magnet to make pictures of the internal organs and blood vessels. It is especially helpful in sickle cell to look for damage to the brain, certain infections, and early bone damage. MRI can look for damage to blood vessels and is now also used to estimate iron levels in the liver, heart, pancreas, kidneys, and other organs.

X-Rays
The clinicians may order X-rays of the chest when looking for pneumonia or acute chest syndrome. Bone X-rays may help diagnose damage due to sickle cells or infection. This is still the fastest and most cost-effective way to look for certain complications.

Bone Scans

Sometimes clinicians cannot tell if an infection is present in the bones. A substance that "lights up" in areas of infection is given by IV, and the scanner traces where the substance goes. If it concentrates in one area of bone, an infection may be found that needs special treatment. Bone scans also help identify bones to repair after infarction due to sickled cells blocking blood vessels to the bone.

Vascular Access Ports (Ports)

Individuals with sickle cell may get a lot of IVs and blood tests done over the years, causing their veins to be scarred and not usable. When healthcare providers must search and stick multiple places just to get blood samples and give medications and fluids, it may be time to consider a port. Ports are plastic catheters put into a large vein in the arm or chest with a small, round, quarter-sized chamber put under the skin. This chamber has a special self-sealing top that can be punctured multiple times by special bent needles. The port gives healthcare providers a quick and reliable access to get blood samples and give IV fluids, blood, and medications.

The good news is that, with the help of such ports, procedures usually require only one needle stick. The bad news is that these ports do not last forever because they become clotted or infected and must be replaced. Clots may require treatment with blood thinners, and infections may require long treatments with antibiotics. This happens more commonly if they are not properly flushed or are improperly cleaned and handled. The port must be flushed with a weak heparin solution at least once a month to prevent blood from clotting within the tubing. The port must be accessed using a sterile technique to keep bacteria from getting into the port and your blood stream. It is good for you to learn all about the sterile technique and the correct needles to use so you can prevent healthcare providers who are not familiar with ports from causing an infection or other complications. Many centers do not use ports for blood drawing to help prevent complications. Even with the best of care, they may clot, become infected, or wear out.

There are now special ports that can be used for chronic exchange transfusions. These are important because it can become very hard to find veins that can support erythrocytaphoresis, exchange using a machine.

IN THE HOSPITAL

If you or a family member needs to be admitted to the hospital, there are some matters that could make the stay more comfortable. In many hospitals, your care may be managed by a hospital-based physician (hospitalist) or a physician extender (physician assistant or nurse practitioner) who is new to you. It is important that you have a care plan from your sickle cell doctor that outlines your past treatments, complications, and present treatment plan. If pain is a major issue, ask for a PCA (patient-controlled analgesia pump), which gives you almost complete control over the timing and dosage of pain medication. Learn how to use the PCA to best control your pain. If PCA is not an option, ask your doctor to use fixed timing of the pain medication, not as needed (PRN) dosing. Combinations of pain medicines may be more effective in controlling your pain and may have fewer side-effects.

Whenever you have pain in the chest or upper stomach, or if you are in bed for more than a day, you should use an incentive spirometer, or "blow bottle." This device exercises the lungs and prevents acute chest syndrome.

Be a teacher. Many nurses and other healthcare providers have not cared for a lot of sickle cell patients. Do some gentle teaching about the disease and its impact on your life. This will help build empathy in the hospital workers. Some of our patients and families find that visiting the nurses on the hospital wards when they feel better and thanking them for their care goes a long way in making them more positive about sickle cell patients.

Keep track of fluids you drink and those you get from an IV, and track how much urine you excrete. The IV fluid of choice is D5W (a 5% solution of dextrose in water, or "sugar water"). This fluid forces water into the dehydrated red blood cells and may reverse the sickling.

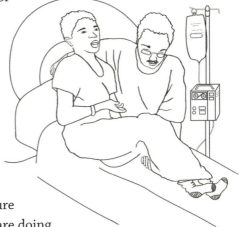

Get out of bed and walk as much as possible if you are able and allowed to do so. Use forms of distraction that you have found reduce your pain. Make sure you tell the providers what you are doing so they do not think your activity is a sign that you're not in pain.

Be sure to ask questions about what is going on, including about your tests and the results. Having someone with you is important, because the medications may make you sleepy and forget what is going on.

Surgery

If you or a family member is scheduled for surgery, here is what you need to know in order make the experience as positive as possible:

- You may need to have a simple blood transfusion to get your hemoglobin to a level of 10 g/dL. Studies have shown that this prevents postoperative complications such as acute chest syndrome. It is best if the transfusion can be given a week or two before the surgery.
- If your hemoglobin is already 10 g/dL or higher, your doctor may want to do an exchange transfusion if you are having major surgery in order to keep your blood from sludging, clotting, and causing complications.
- It is important that you have an IV if you are not going to be allowed to take in fluids by mouth (NPO) for a prolonged time before the surgery.
- Tell the anesthesiologist (the doctor who puts you to sleep for the surgery) that you have sickle cell disease. It is important that you are kept warm, well hydrated, and well oxygenated before, during, and after the surgery to prevent a pain episode.
- You should be placed on an incentive spirometer or blow bottle to exercise your lungs after the surgery. This will help prevent acute chest syndrome.

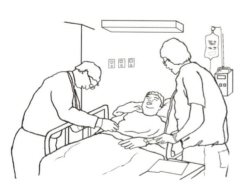

- As soon as permitted, start getting out of bed and walking around to prevent acute chest and blood clots. Follow the nurses' and doctors' directions about this.
- You may need higher doses of pain medicines to control your pain from surgery because of your past

treatments for pain. The doctors and nurses may not be comfortable giving these doses, so you may need to have them consult with your sickle cell doctor about your pain control if there are problems.

INFORMATION TO KEEP

You should keep a mini-medical record of all important complications you have had, your medication allergies, your usual lab values, the pain medications that normally work for you, transfusion reactions and red blood cell antibodies, and your doctor's name and phone number. If you receive transfusions, you should also keep a record of the name and numbers of the hospitals where you have been transfused. It is especially important to carry this information when you travel away from home, where you may have to visit a new hospital. A sample of critical information you should always carry with you is in the resources section. This can be a paper document that you carry with you, sometimes called a medical passport. There are also several smartphone applications that you can use to store this information on your cell phone, like Evernote. You can sign up for registries like "Get Connected" from the Sickle Cell Disease Association of America—visit *www4.gvtsecure.com/reg_scdaa* and click on the "Register" button.

11

Pain Assessment and Pain Management

INTRODUCTION

Of the many symptoms that can torment sickle cell patients, pain is one of the most common and distressing. This chapter tells you what you need to know about:

- The causes of pain;
- Pain prevention;
- Home treatment;
- Emergency treatment; and
- In-patient treatment in the hospital.

We can't repeat it too often: knowledge is power. The more you know about the causes, prevention, and treatment of pain, the better your comfort and the chances of an early recovery. Certain types and causes of pain require a clinician's help and advice about treatment. Until recently, a healthcare professional's assessment of a patient's pain was not done routinely and could be quite subjective. Today, the Joint Commission on Accreditation of Healthcare Organizations (commonly called, simply, "the Joint Commission"), the independent agency that inspects and certifies all US hospitals, has issued new standards for pain assessment, treatment, and education. These new pain management standards should improve the pain care sickle cell patients receive.

In 2015, the National Institutes of Health released new treatment guidelines that included pain management, and in 2016 the Centers for Disease Control issued important guidelines on treatment of chronic pain with opiates. In addition, the Office of the Assistant Secretary for Health at the

US Department of Health and Human Services launched a "National Pain Strategy" to reduce the burden borne by those with chronic pain by developing a system of care where all people receive appropriate, high-quality and evidence-based care for pain. These and many other initiatives should result in improved pain care.

The most common acute problem of sickle cell disease causing presentation for acute treatment is the sickle pain episode (also unfortunately termed a pain "crisis"). A pain episode is defined as "a self-limited episode of diffuse, reversible pain often occurring in the extremities, back, chest, and abdomen." The severity of pain can range from mild attacks of five minutes to excruciating pain lasting days or weeks and requiring hospitalization. This intense pain is believed to be caused by the inflammatory response to bone or marrow death (necrosis), reduced blood flow (ischemia), ischemic muscle, and ischemic bowel, resulting from the obstruction and sludging of blood flow produced by sickled red blood cells (erythrocytes).

Although the pain episode is almost never a cause of death, affected individuals often fear serious complications or death at the time they are in pain.

The frequency of pain episode varies with each person, depending upon his or her hemoglobin phenotype, physical condition, and many other variables. Trigger factors include events that cause increased physical and psychological stress, especially fever, dehydration, overexertion, rapid temperature change, intense joy, or anger. Episodes, however, most frequently occur without any apparent causes.

Recent studies in children and adults show that most acute pain episodes are successfully managed at home by individuals and their families. It is very important for the individual to learn how to manage his or her pain based on the type of pain they are having and the severity of the pain. It is also essential that the individual know when he or she should immediately seek medical care for a pain episode. If fever, other illness, unusual or persistent pain is present, or vomiting that prevents the individual from staying hydrated, they should immediately seek medical care for the pain episode because other, more serious complications may also be present.

The management of a pain episode in a healthcare setting begins with a rapid, complete clinical evaluation to exclude life-threatening complications and identify causes of pain that are not related to sickle cell disease.

A detailed history and physical examination allow the doctor to identify treatable factors such as infection, dehydration, acidosis from any cause, emotional stress, extreme temperature exposure, or ingestion of other substances such as alcohol or recreational drugs.

Because there are no characteristic physical or laboratory findings that occur with or define the severity of a pain episode, the patient's assessment must be accepted. Pain is what the individual experiences and reports.

Treatment of a pain episode at home or in a medical care facility includes hydration, analgesics, rest, and treatment of the underlying causes, such as infection.

RECORDING PAIN

It helps you and your healthcare providers to record the following information about your pain in a daily diary. Use the acronym LOCATES to locate the pain:

L—Location. Note the exact location of the pain, and describe if it "travels" anywhere.

O—Other Symptoms. Record any other symptoms like fever, nausea, or cough that come with the pain.

C—Character. Describe the pain. Is it unusual for them? Deep? Burning? Throbbing? Other?

A—Aggravating and Alleviating Things. What makes the pain better, and what makes the pain worse?

T—Timing. When did the pain start? Has it been there the entire time, or does it come and go?

E—Environment and Effect. Where were you and what were you doing when the pain started? How does the pain affect your daily routine?

S—Severity. You should find a way of measuring and reporting your pain that works for you. You can use words like no pain, mild, moderate or severe; use a number from 0 to 10; or use a paper scale. Pain scales should be available in the ER and the hospital. A scale you should be familiar with is the Visual Analog Scale, or VAS. It is a 10-centimeter line with numbers from 0 to 10. Zero is "no pain," and 10 is "the worst pain you have ever had in your life." Mark on the line where you would rate your level of pain.

Many health systems record your assessment of pain with a number from 0 to 10. There are also scales showing series of faces and colors to help you assess your level of pain.

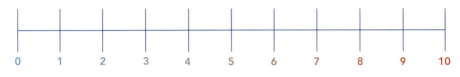

Be consistent and be honest in your report of pain. Overstating your pain score, thinking healthcare providers will otherwise not treat you with enough pain medication, can lead you to being overdosed and having more side effects. Develop a sense of trust with your healthcare providers. They need to believe you to treat your stated level of pain with the appropriate amount of medication.

TYPES OF PAIN

There are at least five identifiable types of pain, each with different treatments.

1. Acute sickle cell pain episode—pain that can last for several minutes to several days, caused by reduced flow from the sickled red blood cells. This pain is usually felt deep in the bones and muscles of the arms, legs, and back. Pain in the head, chest, or belly—or pain with fever—should be immediately evaluated by a healthcare provider.

2. Acute pain from another cause—pain that comes on suddenly and feels different from your usual pain episode should be checked by your healthcare provider. Individuals with sickle cell also get the same pains as those without sickle cell such as headaches, pain from injury, menstrual cramps, appendicitis, stomach cramps, arthritis, slipped discs, and many others.

3. Chronic pain from sickle cell bone damage—pain that lasts longer than a few weeks and may be present daily. This occurs when bones and other structures are damaged by the blocked blood flow.

4. Chronic pain from other causes—daily pain that lasts more than six weeks caused by such things as a slipped disc, rheumatoid arthritis, old injuries, and so forth.

5. Chronic nerve pain—pain caused by damage to the nerves from injury, sickle cell blockage, or other conditions like diabetes. Nerve damage causes a burning, tingling, numbing type of discomfort on a daily basis.

TREATING PAIN

Acute Sickle Cell Pain Episode

If this is a typical pain episode, note the type of pain and then start by drinking more water, lying down, and resting. Taking a warm bath can help, and so can distractions, such as music, TV, a game, or relaxation techniques. Massage to the area may be helpful. You can also try moist heat (from a towel placed in warm water then wrung out).

The best medications to start treatment are nonsteroidal anti-inflammatory drugs (NSAIDs), like ibuprofen (Motrin, Advil) or naproxen (Naprosyn, Aleve). There are many other NSAIDs that may be prescribed by your doctor. They block pain in the muscles and bones and they reduce inflammation that is causing the pain. NSAIDs do not cause drowsiness, and they are good for menstrual cramps. The doses recommended should always be followed because too high a dose causes kidney and liver damage. NSAIDs also have a ceiling effect—that is, higher doses will not provide more pain relief than the recommended dose. NSAIDs should not be used if there are kidney problems, stomach ulcers, bleeding problems, or in certain individuals with asthma. It should be noted that ibuprofen can cause stomach upset and ulcers, so it is best taken after a meal or snack. Ibuprofen can also interfere with the ability of platelets to stop bleeding from cuts.

Acetaminophen (one trade name is Tylenol) also is a good over-the-counter drug for starting pain treatment. However, acetaminophen also blocks fevers, which could indicate a serious life-threatening infection is present, so check with your doctor. You can take acetaminophen at the same time as an NSAID. Acetaminophen is often combined with mild opiates like codeine (Tylenol 3) or hydrocodone (Vicodin) that are available only by prescription. The amount of acetaminophen taken must be limited to recommended guidelines because too much acetaminophen will damage the liver. Acetaminophen also causes liver damage when combined with alcohol even at recommended doses.

Aspirin is a very effective medicine for control of pain. Aspirin has the same cautions as ibuprofen. One particular caution to note is that aspirin has been associated with Reye's syndrome, which has serious effects on the brain and liver, and should not be given to children with fever or cold symptoms.

Codeine, hydrocodone, oxycodone, and hydromorphone are oral opiate medications that block pain in the brain. These medications are usually given in combination with acetaminophen, aspirin, or ibuprofen but can be given by themselves to block pain when a fever is being monitored. They will not block fever or platelets, and they don't cause stomach ulcers. These medications may cause drowsiness, nausea, and itching. They may also cause constipation, so be sure to drink plenty of water and eat plenty of fiber-rich foods like fruit, vegetables, and whole grains when using them. They are available by prescription only. If your healthcare provider has given you other pain medications, these may also be started as prescribed.

When treating your pain at home, start with an NSAID or acetaminophen if you can take these medications. If the pain is controlled with either of these medications, keep taking them as recommended until the pain gets better. You can add acetaminophen to an NSAID if the pain is not controlled to your comfort level. You can then add an oral opioid that has been prescribed by the doctor. Continue the NSAID or acetaminophen if there is none in the pill with the opioid. Stop taking them separately if they are in a combination with the opioid. If you can't control your pain with these methods, it is time to see your doctor or go to the emergency room.

Acute Pain From Another Cause
Pain in the head, chest, or abdomen and pain with fever should be evaluated; then the pain can be safely managed. You can manage pain from menstrual cramps, simple headaches, and small injuries like anyone without sickle cell.

Chronic Pain From Sickle Cell Bone Damage
The best treatment for this type of pain is not based on use of pain medications but physical means such as heat and rest. Avoid activities that make the pain worse. The goal of treatment is not complete removal of the pain, because this is almost never possible all of the time. Rather, the goal is to reduce pain to a level that is tolerable and that improves quality of life and daily functioning. Strategies include change in behavior, physical therapy, weight loss, carrying less weight, injections or transcutaneous electrical nerve simulators (TENS) if the pain is localized, and mild heat.

PAIN MEDICATIONS AVAILABLE WITHOUT PRESCRIPTION

Name	Dosage by Weight	Notes
Acetaminophen (Tylenol)	20 lbs. → 100 mg 30 lbs. → 150 mg 40 lbs. → 200 mg 50 lbs. → 250 mg 60 lbs. → 300 mg 70 lbs. → 350 mg 80 lbs. → 400 mg 90 lbs. → 450 mg 100 lbs. → 500 mg 120 lbs.+ → 650 mg	➡ Use every 4 hours ➡ Will block fever ➡ Will not upset stomach ➡ Does not block inflammation ➡ Maximum adult dose 4,000 mg in 24 hours ➡ Toxic doses damage the liver ➡ May damage the kidneys and liver in chronic high doses
Ibuprofen (Advil, Motrin)	20 lbs. → 100 mg 30 lbs. → 150 mg 40 lbs. → 200 mg 50 lbs. → 250 mg 60 lbs. → 300 mg 70 lbs. → 350 mg 80 lbs. → 400 mg 90 lbs. → 450 mg 100 lbs. → 500 mg 120 lbs.+ → 600 mg	➡ Use every 6 to 8 hours ➡ Will block fever ➡ May cause stomach ulcers ➡ Blocks inflammation ➡ Maximum adult dose 3,200 mg in 24 hours ➡ May increase blood pressure
Aspirin	Adults only 625 mg every 4-6 hrs. 80 mg per day to slow clotting	➡ All of the same notes as ibuprofen ➡ May cause Reye's syndrome in children—do not use in children

NSAIDs are very good for this type of pain because inflammation is usually present. Long-acting arthritis medications are very helpful for daily pain control. For long-term use, salsalate, Celebrex (celecoxib), and Mobic (meloxicam) may be safer for the stomach and duodenum than other arthritis medications because they are associated with fewer erosions and ulcers. You should be aware that there are now some serious concerns about several of the NSAIDs in that, if taken frequently, they may increase the risk of stroke and heart attack.

Opioid medications may be used with the NSAIDs for very short periods if the pain is not controlled, or alone if the NSAIDs cannot be used. However, opioids appear to cause more harm than good when they are given for long periods for chronic pain. You and your providers should read the information available on the CDC website before considering using opioids for chronic pain. (*www.cdc.gov/drugoverdose/prescribing/guideline.html*). All opioids block pain in the brain and cause drowsiness, constipation, tolerance problems, physical dependence, and physical withdrawal if they are suddenly stopped. A stool softener to prevent constipation should be used when opiates are being taken daily.

Certain antidepressant and seizure medications may also help fight chronic pain. Tricyclic antidepressant medication, such as amitriptyline or certain serotonin reuptake inhibitors, may work in combination with pain medication to help fight chronic pain. Neurontin (gabapentin) and Lyrica (pregabalin) may also be helpful if there is a neuropathic component. (See "Chronic Nerve Pain or Neuropathic Pain"). Muscle relaxants can help to reduce painful muscle spasm.

Chronic Pain from Other Causes
All of the previous therapies listed are used to control chronic pain from causes other than sickle cell disease, as are nerve blocks and disease-specific medications.

Chronic Nerve Pain or Neuropathic Pain
Treatment with seizure medication, such as gabapentin and pregabalin, has been helpful in control of neuropathic pain. Studies in patients with diabetic neuropathic pain suggest that tricyclic antidepressant medications, such as amitriptyline or certain serotonin and norepinephrine reuptake inhibitors (SNRIs) and selective serotonin reuptake inhibitors (SSRIs) are also useful

for this type of pain. These antidepressants appear to have a direct effect on chronic pain. They may also provide additional benefits in improving pain if there is an element of depression that is very common in individuals with chronic pain.

IN THE EMERGENCY ROOM

The emergency room (ER) is the next stop if home treatment fails or if there are danger signs such as:

- fever;
- weakness;
- atypical pain;
- headache;
- chest pain; and/or
- abdominal pain.

Special emergency rooms for sickle cell patients, often called day hospitals or infusion centers, are becoming more common in major cities across the country. Some medical centers are establishing extended care units within the emergency room for problems like sickle pain episodes. At present, most sickle cell patients still receive care for their pain episodes in the nearest emergency room. Some hospitals may not have ER staff members who are well trained in the care of sickle cell patients. The best defense is a good offense—come prepared with knowledge.

What Should Happen

Here, in a nutshell, is what you should expect when you go into an emergency room:

- First, you should be seen promptly within 30 minutes of arriving. Your vital signs should be taken, including your temperature (normal: 98.6°F/37°C or below), breathing rate (normal: 15–20 breaths per minute); heart rate (pulse; normal: 60–100 beats per minute at rest), blood pressure (normal: 90/60–120/80 mmHg at rest), pulse oximetry (a measure of the oxygen in your red blood cells; normal: 95%–100%), and your pain intensity score (how much pain you are having, from 0 to 10).
- A nurse should ask you about your main problem and assess how quickly you will be seen. In all emergency rooms, the most critical conditions must be seen first. A pain episode is not life-threaten-

ing, but there are symptoms that could require immediate treatment, such as fever, chills, headache, chest pain, abdominal pain, weakness, and abdominal swelling.
- A doctor, physician assistant, or nurse practitioner should examine you for signs of infection or complications. He or she should look in your ears, eyes, mouth, and nose, and listen to your heart, chest, and abdomen. He or she should also feel your abdomen for tenderness or swelling of the liver or spleen, and should check all of the areas that are hurting for swelling, heat, or tenderness.
- Blood may be drawn for tests, including a complete blood count (CBC), reticulocyte count, and chemistry values. A urine sample may be checked for blood, protein, and infection.
- Your doctor may have developed an individual treatment plan for you. Generally, an IV should be started with D5W and saline (salt) in water to rehydrate the sickled red blood cells. In most cases, normal saline should not be used.
- Pain medication should be given through the IV if possible, and on a fixed time schedule based on the medication. Giving medication on a fixed schedule assures a good pain-fighting blood level can be reached and kept. If pain medication is given as needed or as requested, the pain relief is like a roller coaster going up and down. Pain medication given by a patient-controlled analgesia (PCA) pump allows a continuous amount to go in all the time. You can use the pump button to give extra doses at a safe rate for extra pain control. Your pain should be reassessed periodically to see if the medication is working.
- Try to continue distraction therapy by reading a book, watching TV, listening to music, or playing a game. Relaxation techniques can be used.

Common Medications Used in Emergency Rooms

Many good pain medications are available for pain episodes, and many work better in combinations. (Note: There are dangers associated with pain medication use, and it is essential to carefully consider the risks of using prescription opioids alongside their benefits.) Among those frequently used are the following:

- *Morphine*. Morphine is an opiate that blocks pain in the brain.

It can be given by mouth, IV, in a PCA pump, or by a shot in the muscle. Morphine takes effect in fifteen minutes and lasts up to three hours. It slows breathing down as the dose goes up. It can cause itching, nausea, vomiting, and constipation. The body can become physically dependent on morphine for several days after use. In coming off of morphine, the dose should be tapered off and not stopped suddenly.

- *Nalbuphine (Nubain).* Nalbuphine is an injectable pain medication that is safe and effective in controlled doses. It does not slow respiration as morphine does. Nalbuphine has a "ceiling effect," so if it does not control pain as required, you must switch to another medication. This medication has fewer side effects, with less itching, nausea, and drowsiness than morphine. Nalbuphine may cause withdrawal symptoms and it should not be used in individuals taking daily opiates.
- *Ketorolac (Toradol).* This is an IV-administered, nonsteroidal anti-inflammatory drug that blocks pain in the bone and muscle tissue where the blocked blood flow from sickled red cells has caused damage. All of the cautions are the same as for ibuprofen. This medication can only be used for a maximum of five days continuously, or in short courses repeated frequently, because of risk of kidney damage and renal failure.
- *Meperidine (Demerol).* This opiate pain medication is good for acute pain, but not for pain lasting more than a few days. Very few sickle cell programs recommend use of meperidine because of serious side effects. It breaks down in the body to a substance that is a stimulant that causes irritability, and it can cause seizures in high doses. Many hospital and outpatient pharmacies have also stopped stocking the drug. This medication has all of the same cautions as morphine, which is a much better first-choice opiate.
- *Hydromorphone (Dilaudid)* is a potent, fast-acting opioid that is used in many emergency rooms to treat sickle cell disease. It has similar side effects to morphine. Doses are much lower than morphine.
- *Hydroxyzine (Vistaril).* In proper doses, hydroxyzine can prevent nausea and itching caused by opiates. It can also help calm fear.

♦ *Antihistamines (e.g. Benadryl)* can increase the sedation and respiratory depression caused by opioids.

TOLERANCE TO OPIOIDS

All opioid medications become less effective when used regularly to control pain. The brain and nervous system adjust to the medications so that it takes more of it to get the same amount of pain relief. This is called tolerance. Many individuals with sickle cell require much higher doses of opioids to get pain relief than others (such as maternity or surgery patients) because they have received the medications before. Tolerance can become a problem when high doses of opioids are taken for a long period of time, because it becomes impossible to control pain without serious side-effects, which sometimes include the medications actually making the pain worse. This is why opioids are not a good choice for chronic pain and why treatment should be stopped as soon as it is practical.

PHYSICAL DEPENDENCY ON OPIOIDS

All individuals who are given opiates continuously for a period of time will have symptoms of withdrawal if the medications are reduced or stopped rapidly. This is called physical dependency and develops within a week or two of continuous opioid use. If any of the opiate medications are used for several days and then stopped, the body will have withdrawal symptoms such as anxiety, agitation, abdominal cramps, muscle aches, increased tearing, insomnia, irritability, runny nose, sweating, and yawning. Withdrawal may also another sickle cell crisis. This condition can be avoided by slowly decreasing the amount of the medication used over several days to allow the body to adjust. This is why, if opioids are needed for more than a week to control pain, they should not be stopped abruptly but be tapered over about the same period of time they were given for pain control.

DRUG ADDICTION

Drug addiction is a complex behavior related to the use of drugs on a regular basis to achieve effects not related to their primary effect of reducing pain. The diagnosis is difficult in someone with chronic pain or recurrent acute pain. True drug addiction can be diagnosed by the presence of a number of behavior characteristics including, but not limited to, devoting significant amounts of time and energy into compulsively seeking the medications; using the drugs for relief of anxiety or depression, or to get a high; and taking the medication when it is known to be harmful. True drug addiction occurs in 5%–25% of patients seen in primary care on daily opiates. At the Georgia Comprehensive Sickle Cell Center, we followed more than 2,400 sickle cell patients, and only about 5% met the standard for drug addiction. It is very important that these individuals be identified and receive proper treatment for their addiction, because they will suffer needlessly and also reflect negatively on others with sickle cell disease.

There is also two conditions we call "pseudo-addiction." The first is in individuals who are undertreated with opiates and experience uncontrolled pain. Because they are in constant pain, they are appropriately constantly asking for more medication, and healthcare workers mislabel these patients as "addicts with drug-seeking behavior." The second is where an opioid is rapidly tapered or stopped after prolonged use and the individual experiences withdrawal because they have developed physical dependency. Every two to three days they experience a new "pain crisis" and need treatment again. This is treated by tapering the opioid over time so they will not go through withdrawal symptoms.

Until more sickle cell centers are available, patients with pain must keep returning to the ER for help.

ADMISSION TO THE HOSPITAL

Admission to the hospital for more pain management or treatment is recommended within 48 hours of previous therapy, under the following conditions:

- if the pain does not decrease to a manageable level after 8–12 hours of treatment in the ER; and/or
- if a complication is present. That is, if you are experiencing a pain episode with any of the following:
  - infection;
  - temperature over 100.4°F/38°C;
  - pneumonia;
  - kidney infection;
  - blood infection (sepsis);
  - low blood oxygen or too much acid in the blood;
  - stroke;
  - pregnancy;
  - heart problems or failure;
  - priapism that will not go away;
  - blood clots in the lung;

- decrease in blood counts; or
- liver inflammation, gallstones, or gallbladder inflammation.

AS AN INPATIENT

After you are admitted into the hospital, treatment started in the ER should continue. A PCA pump should usually be started for pain control. There are several things you can do to ensure adequate pain management:

- Let the staff know your pain intensity level as a number from 0 to 10. Be honest and consistent, so the staff can provide appropriate treatment.
- Tell the nurses if you are having side effects like nausea, vomiting, constipation, itching, trouble breathing, or feeling drowsy.
- Use an incentive spirometer frequently to prevent acute chest syndrome. A good rule is to take a couple of breaths during each TV ad.
- Get up and walk if you can to prevent blood clots.
- Report your mood to the nursing staff. Feelings of depression, fear, anger, and sadness can all hinder your pain treatment. Counsel from chaplains, social workers, and nurses, as well as medication, can help in many cases.
- Be respectful and do not lash out at doctors, nurses, or other staff. Remember and follow the Golden Rule: treat others as you would want them to treat you.
- Medication by PCA pump is one of the best options for pain control in the hospital. Report to your nurse any change in symptoms, or sites of pain.
- Visiting and thanking the staff after you recover can go a long way in improving your and other patients' care. They will at least know what a wonderful person you are when you are feeling well.

RELAXATION TECHNIQUES

Pain can be helped by thinking about something else. Dwelling on the pain can make it feel worse. Being tense tightens muscles, reduces blood flow, and increases pain. Relaxation techniques help you relax muscles and get your mind off of the pain.

Start by getting in a quiet room, with some soothing music if it is available. Get in a comfortable position. Make a fist, release your fingers, and concentrate on letting them go limp. Tense your arm muscles, and then let them go limp. Tense your shoulders then let them go limp. Tense your neck then let it go limp. "Squench" your face muscles, and let them go limp. Tense your toes and feet, and then let them go limp. Tense your leg muscles, and let them go limp. Tense your stomach, and let it go limp.

At this stage, all of your muscles should be more relaxed. If any feel tense, repeat, tightening and letting the tense muscles go until they are relaxed. Think of a calm place that you have visited, like a beach or park. Meditate on your favorite scriptures, song, or event. Biofeedback, yoga, meditation, and hypnosis are other ways to help you to relax.

CONCLUSION

Discuss your pain-management plan with your healthcare provider when you are well and not in pain. Make a plan that is right for you. Keep this plan with you, after filling in the important information, to share with each healthcare provider you see.

There are free, problem-oriented guidelines for sickle syndromes available for healthcare providers on the Internet 24 hours a day at the Sickle Cell Information Center at *www.scinfo.org*.

12

Managing Depression and Anxiety

People are at their best when each area of their lives is in a healthy balance. A steady decline in one's mood is evidence of depression. This can happen when facing the complications and pain of sickle cell disease. This low state of mood affects the body, the psychological and social state, and the spiritual outlook. Everyone, at some time in his or her life, experiences varying levels of negative feelings in mood due to internal and external issues or concerns; people can be sad and down for a brief time. However, people who experience disturbances in the mood that result in a severe and ongoing clinical depression require immediate attention and professional help, as well as positive support of available family and friends.

Fear or anxiety is a powerful emotion that causes the body to become charged to "run or fight." Constant fear can be harmful to the body, causing stress-related illnesses and even pain events. Naturally, people who live with daily pain often experience mood problems such as anxiety and stress, insomnia, and depression. If chronic pain limits your ordinary activity, the problem can be even worse.

Some studies suggest that chronic pain causes the same changes in brain function as those brought on by stress. The body reacts to stress by putting out stress hormones such as adrenaline. Such hormones allow our hearts to beat faster and our responses to be quicker when we need to cope with, or flee from, danger. In times of chronic stress, such as stress brought on by chronic pain, our bodies continue to put out more stress hormones than usual, even though there is no sudden danger from which we must run.

Constant increased amounts of stress hormones affect our bodies in a variety of ways. These hormones also can affect the mind. When you're stressed or in constant pain, your body doesn't produce enough serotonin, a chemical that helps to regulate several essential functions, such as sleep, mood, and anxiety. When you don't have enough serotonin, you are less able to fight depression and, as some investigators believe, to deal with pain. That is why it's no surprise that people with chronic lower back pain are three to four times more likely to experience depression.

Depression can affect people with chronic pain in more than one way. Studies report the following:

- People in pain who are depressed are more likely to rate their pain as more severe than are people who aren't depressed.
- When depression is accompanied by sleeplessness, people experience more pain, fatigue, and other physical symptoms, as well as depression.
- People with chronic pain and depression more frequently have suicidal thoughts and attempts than people with other chronic medical problems.

Chronically depressed people often don't know that they're depressed. That's why it's so important to be evaluated by your physician, who can determine whether depression is complicating your chronic pain situation. Treating the depression may help improve some of the pain symptoms. *It is urgent that you seek help if you have thoughts of helplessness or of harming yourself or others.*

WHAT ARE THE SYMPTOMS OF SEVERE DEPRESSION?

It is helpful to consider what happens to the whole person when attempting to identify troublesome areas of our lives. A holistic approach is exploring the components of the body, soul, and spirit. The body is composed of the physical areas of concern. The soul area is composed of the mind, will, emotional, and intellectual components that are involved in social relationships and environmental situations. The spirit is associated with the area of the inner being that is often connected with religious beliefs. Unhealthy balances are described in the following areas:

Body/physical disturbances in severe depression include:

- sleeping too much or too little;

- having trouble falling asleep;
- waking up early and not being able to go back to sleep or get up;
- eating too much or too little;
- lacking pleasure in things you ordinarily like to do;
- lacking any fun in life; and
- withdrawing from normal life activities.

Soul/psychosocial disturbances that may be involved in severe depression are:

- life disruptions, such as job change or loss, family changes, and relocation;
- problems with yourself, such as poor self-esteem, anger, shame, anxiety, increased self-destructive or suicidal thoughts, and an inability to concentrate; or
- problems with other people due to one's anger, irritability, arguments, social withdrawal, abuse, neglect, and/or excessive, extended grief.

Spiritual disturbances associated with depression can be:

- guilt and self-pity;
- fear;
- feelings of hopelessness;
- excessive worrying;
- isolation and loneliness;
- feelings of rejection, inferiority, and worthlessness; and
- feeling overburdened or unforgiving.

WHAT ARE SOME TREATMENTS TO CONQUER DEPRESSION?

The good news is that there are ways to return to a healthy balance in all areas in your life and even achieve higher levels of improvement. The following are some suggestions that can help with depression of the body, soul, and spirit.

Healthy Body Balance

Treatments for depression have also proved helpful in also improving pain in those with both chronic pain and depression. Group programs, run by nurses with specialties in pain management, have been found to be successful. Such programs work without medicines, instead emphasizing education and behavior changes. Studies have shown that such programs reduce suffering and improve a sense of well being even for people who have experienced pain for many years.

Besides joining a support group, you may also want to see a therapist (psychologist or psychiatrist). Chronic pain sufferers continually experience the losses that go along with daily pain as well as the accompanying physical changes. A therapist can often be helpful by encouraging you to look at these losses closely and to learn to cope with your feelings about them.

If your depression does not respond to cognitive and behavioral approaches or counseling, or these are not available to you, there are effective medications to treat major depression. Many of these also directly reduce chronic pain. If your physician recommends an antidepressant, understand that he or she is not telling you that your pain is "all in your head." The doctor is offering you an important tool for treating your pain holistically. Many studies show that, even in people who aren't depressed, their chronic headaches, low-back pain, or diabetes-related neuropathic (nerve-ending injury) pain can be lessened through the use of certain antidepressants.

Commonly used antidepressants for pain treatment include older tricyclic antidepressants, such as nortriptyline or amitriptyline. The best dose varies from person to person, and your physician will adjust your dosages to ensure that you are taking the amount that works best for you. These medications are very effective, but they have many side effects you should discuss with your physician before starting.

It is still unclear how effective the newer classes of antidepressants (selective serotonin reuptake inhibitors, or SSRIs) are in improving pain. Some studies have shown improvement, while others have not. There is some evidence that venlafaxine is at least as effective as the older nortriptyline class, with fewer side effects. Certain serotonin and norepinephrine reuptake inhibitor antidepressants (SSNRIs) such as duloxetine have been shown to improve chronic pain caused by nerve damage in individuals with diabetic neuropathy. More work is needed to prove this in sickle cell, but, if one has chronic pain and is depressed, using tricyclic antidepressants or SSNRIs to treat the depression seems very reasonable.

Other things you can do include the following:

- Have a medical checkup to make sure nothing else is wrong when

there is a radical change in physical functioning.
- Follow the medical plan and treatment of medical illness/disease, with laboratory and specialty consultations as needed.
- Get appropriate and supervised pain management by specialists with expertise in chronic pain and sickle cell disease.
- Have dietary and nutritional consultations and support to maintain optimal physical functioning.
- Report and discuss any new symptoms that may arise.
- Get your proper rest, relaxation, sleep, and exercise.

Healthy Soul Balance

Balancing your soul involves three parts:

1. THE "PHASE OF LIFE" BALANCE
- Attend to your needs and the needs of others as they come up so that they do not accumulate and become overwhelming.
- Obtain appropriate counseling support when you need help.
- Identify sources of support for new circumstances.

2. THE RELATIONSHIP WITH YOURSELF
- Realistically identify your positive strengths and weaknesses, obtaining objective assistance if you are unable to do so without help.
- Spend quiet time with yourself so that negative feelings are not suppressed and ignored.
- Do something positive to deal with disturbing feelings and behaviors.
- Get immediate professional help and support from others who care about you whenever you begin to contemplate passive or active suicidal thoughts, plans, or intent.
- Seek help if you are advised to by caring family and friends, even if you cannot see the need yet. Trust their judgment, especially when you know that you are not feeling right.
- Monitor your attitude, behavior, and habits, and keep them positive.
- Cease any behaviors that are abusive or neglectful of yourself or others. Do not be afraid to ask for help, or get help, when another advises you to do so.

3. YOUR RELATIONSHIPS WITH OTHERS

- Establish an active and positive support system.
- Avoid arguments, and strive for effective and positive communication.
- Settle disagreements quickly, and take accountability and responsibility for any problems you have caused.
- Maintain social contacts for support, recreation, and companionship.
- Terminate any abusive or neglectful behaviors by another person. Do not be afraid to ask for help to do so.
- Talk to someone you trust when your grieving does not seem to get better or it seems to be getting worse. Get help if a loved one or colleague tells you that your grief is worsening.

Healthy Spirit Balance

Easing depression is the treatment for both the body and soul, but your spirit needs tending to as well. Some suggestions to raise your spirits include the following:

- Monitor your attitudes and behavior, and do the "right" things—not violating spiritual guidelines, disciplines, or principles.
- Ask for spiritual support and guidance when you need it, such as times of struggle with helplessness, hopelessness, worry, fear, heaviness, or rejection.
- Accept spiritual support and fellowship from your community resources.
- Maintain a positive outlook. During times of distress and trouble, find hope through prayer, friendships, spiritual gathering, music, videos, etc.
- Focus on solutions, not problems.
- Practice being patient when going through difficult circumstances.
- Maintain the positives in where you go, with whom you spend time, and what you spend your time doing.
- Seek out situations, environments, and people that increase your sense of security, safety, and support. Strive to be such a resource to others as well.
- Sing and listen to uplifting music.
- Practice fun hobbies and activities.

- Review and meditate on encouraging reading material, programs, plays, etc.
- Avoid talking negatively with others. Seek to maintain peacefulness.
- Avoid dwelling on thoughts and situations that bring fretting, fear, or anxiety.
- Maintain a thankful attitude for life.
- Avoid and/or terminate bad relationships, but cultivate those that promote love, compassion, understanding, accountability, responsibility, and growth.
- Seek wise spiritual counsel, helpers, and encouragers to get help during spiritual distress.
- Avoid situations that promote debt, fighting and arguments, divisions, and doubt.
- Set growth goals that get your thinking and behavior out of dysfunctional past behaviors, that are progressively achievable, and that keep you being the best that you are meant to be.

ANXIETY

Anxiety, which is bad enough all by itself, can also increase pain. The ability to feel "in control" of the situation can influence the degree of pain you experience. The more you know about what is causing your pain and how you can best control it, the less your anxiety and pain.

Because they know that anxiety makes pain worse, doctors often prescribe anti-anxiety medications for people with chronic pain. Medications commonly used to control anxiety can be very dangerous when combined with opioids. Tranquilizers in the benzodiazepine class SHOULD NOT be taken with opioids; in addition, they have their own dependency problems. Non-pharmacological approaches such as counseling, meditation, music therapy, massage therapy, relaxation techniques, cognitive and behavioral approaches and other psychological approaches are most important.

If these do not work, medications may be added carefully. Antihistamines and antidepressants with anti-anxiety actions can be considered. Antihistamines such as diphenhydramine or hydroxyzine have anti-anxiety effects without posing dependence problems. Drowsiness is a possible side effect with either group. If strong medications are used, a psychiatrist who also treats pain needs to be involved in their management.

13

Hydroxyurea and Glutamine Therapy

Hemoglobin F (fetal hemoglobin) directly interferes with the clumping together of sickle hemoglobin in red blood cells and prevents sickling, even better than hemoglobin A does. Between conception and birth, our predominant hemoglobin is hemoglobin F. After birth, the level of fetal hemoglobin falls. Infants with sickle cell disease do not usually have apparent problems until after about six months of age, when the levels of hemoglobin F have fallen substantially. Having a high percentage of circulating hemoglobin F protects against sickling and its many complications. Individuals with higher hemoglobin F live longer, have fewer pain episodes, and run a higher total hemoglobin level.

The drug hydroxyurea has proven effective in raising the percentage of hemoglobin F by stimulating the production of protective fetal hemoglobin within the red cells. Studies done twenty years ago show that adult patients on hydroxyurea have 50% fewer pain episodes, fewer episodes of acute chest episodes, 50% fewer blood transfusions, and 50% less need for hospitalization. Several studies in children have shown efficacy and short-term safety and no bad effects on the child's growth and development. A recent study in very young children confirmed benefits in children that were equal to those found in adults. A number of studies are suggesting that individuals with sickle cell anemia and sickle thalassemia who are on hydroxyurea are living longer than those not taking the drug.

The benefits of hydroxyurea are:

- decreased frequency and severity of pain crises;
- decreased frequency and severity of acute chest syndrome;

- ♦ decreased need for blood transfusions;
- ♦ protection of brain functioning;
- ♦ longer life span;
- ♦ less priapism; and
- ♦ possible weight gain.

For these and other reasons, an expert panel made a public statement in 2008 that hydroxyurea deserves to be more widely used for sickle cell treatment.[1] The NIH Guidelines recommend use of hydroxyurea and provide guidelines for its administration.[2]

But there are also restrictions to its use. Because hydroxyurea, like other strong medications, has potential side effects, its use is reserved for sickle cell patients with the most problems. Its safety for use in children with sickle cell anemia is now supported by many studies, and it was officially approved by the FDA for use in children in 2017.

All available brands of hydroxyurea contain some lactose as filler. About 70% of African Americans and a similar percentage of other groups prone to sickle cell anemia are lactose intolerant after childhood. Reactions may include bloating, increased intestinal gas, and diarrhea and nausea that can be controlled by giving lactase with the medication.

Although hydroxyurea causes birth defects in lab rodents, birth defects have not been seen in human babies born to parents taking this drug; however, people on hydroxyurea must plan to avoid conceiving children by using contraception or abstinence while taking this treatment. Discuss a strategy with your doctor for stopping hydroxyurea if you are planning a child. Hydroxyurea is present in the breast milk of women taking the drug, so nursing women should avoid using it.

Because hydroxyurea may also cause genetic changes in developing sperm cells and a decrease in sperm count, men should not take hydroxyurea for at least three months before attempting conception with their partners.

Hydroxyurea reduces the numbers of red blood cells, white blood cells, and platelets being made by the bone marrow. While you are taking hydroxyurea, your blood counts need to be checked frequently to make sure they are not too low. Hydroxyurea should be stopped if:

---

1 *consensus.nih.gov/2008/sicklecellstatement.htm*
2 *www.nhlbi.nih.gov/health-pro/guidelines/sickle-cell-disease-guidelines*

- your total white blood cell count is less than 2,500, because this could seriously reduce your ability to resist infection;
- your platelet count is below 100,000, because this could increase your risk of serious bleeding; or
- you have severe anemia, because your red blood cell count and hemoglobin could fall too low and your vital organs not receive enough oxygen.

Once your counts have recovered it should be restarted, often at a lower dose.

Apart from the possible side effects already discussed, less severe, but more frequent, side effects reported in people taking hydroxyurea include:

- gastrointestinal disturbances;
- rashes;
- weight gain;
- hair loss;
- darkening of toenails and fingernails;
- bleeding not due to low platelet counts; and
- an increased frequency of infection.

There were concerns about leukemia risk, but new data shows that hydroxyurea use in sickle cell and other types of blood diseases is not linked to a higher risk of leukemia.

LABORATORY TESTS YOU SHOULD HAVE BEFORE STARTING HYDROXYUREA

Before starting hydroxyurea, patients should have the following laboratory tests done:

- complete blood count, which includes hemoglobin, hematocrit, white blood cells, and platelets
- liver function and kidney function tests.

These tests need to be repeated frequently during therapy.

Hydroxyurea needs to be taken every day for it to be effective. The hydroxyurea dose is usually started low and increased if the blood counts remain high enough. Once the highest dose is found that does not cause the counts to get low, this is called the maximum tolerated dose (MTD) and continued. If the counts get too low, the hydroxyurea is stopped to allow the low cell counts to come back up to a safe level; the drug is then restarted at a lower dose.

The full benefit of hydroxyurea can take up to three or four months to reach. It is very important to give it a chance before stopping it. Not taking hydroxyurea regularly is the most common reason it does not work.

MONITORING HYDROXYUREA

Complete blood counts must be done at least every two weeks while the MTD is being found. If the counts remain in an acceptable range, then the dose may be increased every six to 12 weeks over 24 consecutive weeks until the highest tolerated dose (35 mg/kg/day) is reached. Once the blood counts are stable, they are usually checked every month. The frequency of monitoring can be decreased further if blood counts are stable. Because hydroxyurea is mostly eliminated from the body by the kidneys, the dose often has to be reduced and monitoring has to be more frequent in those with impaired kidney function. Details of management are provided in the NIH Guidelines.

Hydroxyurea has helped many with sickle cell anemia and sickle β^0 thalassemia regain near-normal lives. All individuals with these types of sickle cell disease should consider taking hydroxyurea. The benefits in those with Hb SC disease and sickle β^+ thalassemia are less clear. Check with your healthcare provider to see if it might be an option for you. Like all medications, it may take a while to find the best dosage with the least side effects for your body. It also takes a number of months to know how well it will work for you. If you start hydroxyurea, take it every day as directed and take it for at least four to six months before deciding it is not working for you.

GLUTAMINE

L-glutamine oral powder is a new medication for sickle cell disease. It was approved by the FDA in 2017 and first entered the US market in 2018 under the brand name Endari.

Glutamine is an amino acid. It is part of the food protein that we eat. Glutamine works primarily by boosting the antioxidant properties of the red blood cell. Antioxidants help the body minimize oxidant damage. Oxidant damage is the same thing that causes iron to rust and sliced apples and avocados to turn brown, and in the human body it increases the risk of cancer, heart disease, and stroke. Sickled red cells have more oxidant damage than other red cells. By boosting the antioxidant properties in red blood cells, glutamine helps the body fight oxidant damage and cut down on inflammation.

Glutamine may help make sickle cell disease milder. People in the clinical research studies on glutamine had fewer pain episodes (by 25%), fewer hospital days (by 25%), and less acute chest syndrome (by half). It does not cure sickle cell disease.

A benefit of glutamine is that it appears to be safe, and only one out of ten people participating in trials prior to FDA approval had any side effects at all. The side effects that were reported include constipation, gurgle noises from the stomach, nausea, and chest tightness. Regular blood tests to monitor organ functions are not needed for patients on glutamine.

Glutamine that is used as medication has been purified and comes in packets of powder, each about half the size of a packet of hot chocolate mix. Stir the powder in a drink or food like water, juice, milk, applesauce, or yogurt. Glutamine is usually taken twice a day, but be sure to take the number of packets prescribed by your doctor as directed.

FREQUENTLY ASKED QUESTIONS ABOUT GLUTAMINE THERAPY

What is the cost of Endari? Is it covered by insurance?
Like all medicine, the cost of Endari depends on your insurance carrier. The specialty pharmacy will help identify the cost in your situation. Endari prescription gets covered by insurance on a case-by-case basis. So far our experience is about 85% approval rate. There can be some co-payment.

Can Endari be taken with hydroxyurea?
Yes, the clinical research was actually mostly done with people already on hydroxyurea, and adding the Endari helped them have milder sickle cell course.

Can Endari be taken during pregnancy?
Ask your doctor. There is no theoretical reason that should be a problem, but we don't have any specific experience to show you.

Does it interfere with any of my other medicines?
Ask your doctor. In the clinical research available as of late 2018, Endari was given to people taking many different medicines for sickle cell and no problems were found so far. There is no theoretical reason that should be a problem, but we don't have any specific experience to show you.

What is the difference between Endari and glutamine available over the counter at vitamin stores?
Endari is available only by prescription and might be covered by insurance. Endari is more purified and its production is regulated and more supervised than food supplements are.

What do most people mix Endari into?
Applesauce, water, and juice seem to be the most popular. One family found that taking Endari with hamburger increased nausea. Be sure to choose something cold—you don't want to put Endari into something so hot that it cooks the powder.

Should I take it when I am in the hospital with pain?
You can if you want to take it during typical pain. You might need to bring your supply from home. Ask your doctor. If you are in the ICU or you cannot take oral medicines, the Endari will be stopped.

Is it a natural product? Is it a meat product?
Endari is a natural product made from sugar cane. It is not a meat product.

Bone Marrow Transplantation

KEONE'S STORY

Keone Penn underwent the world's first unrelated cord blood transplant for sickle cell disease at Children's Healthcare of Atlanta at Egleston on December 11, 1998. Keone had been receiving monthly blood transfusions at Grady ever since he had a stroke at age 5. He had been coming regularly to the hospital ever since. At the age of 24, Keone became a pioneer. Keone did not have a brother or sister match to donate non-sickle bone marrow, so the next logical step was to use an unrelated donor's blood stem cells from

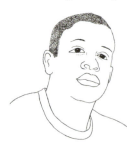

umbilical cord blood. Blood stem cells are very early cells that can produce every kind of blood cell when growing in the bone marrow.

Keone opened the door for the many sickle cell patients who do not have a sibling match but who have enough complications to merit the risk of the procedure. Twelve years after the transplant, Keone was free of sickle cell, but was still battling a number of complications, including the donor cells' attack on his tissues (a problem called graft-versus-host disease). Keone and his family were brave pioneers in the quest for a cure that may someday be available to all of those with sickle cell disease. Keone died in 2013 at the age of 27, the victim of an assault.

TRANSPLANTS: A PROBLEMATIC CURE

In addition to the treatments discussed, a cure for sickle cell anemia already actually exists. That cure is bone marrow transplantation (BMT). You might wonder why, if there is a cure, doctors still treat the disease with treatments that do not cure.

There are two answers to that. First, suitable bone marrow donors are not easy to find. Second, bone marrow transplantation is a risky proposition itself. For sickle cell patients who have a matched sibling donor, the risk of death from the transplant procedure is about 5%, and there is also risk of serious infections, rejection, and graft-versus-host disease.

Furthermore, the donor runs risks with anesthesia and blood loss; these are much smaller risks, but they are still real. However, newer methods allow stem cells for transplant to be collected from the blood of the donor using apheresis, reducing the risk to the donor.

The high cost of bone marrow transplantation and follow-up care must also be considered.

MATCHING TISSUE TYPES

For the usual type of transplant, the donor and recipient must be closely matched in tissue type (also called human leukocyte antigen [HLA] type). In general, the closer the two tissue types resemble each other, the better the chance of a successful transplantation. HLA testing is done on a blood sample drawn from the donor and recipient. Differing blood types (red blood cell incompatibility) is not a barrier to successful bone marrow transplantation as it is for blood transfusion. An HLA-matched brother or sister, if available, is the best choice as a bone marrow donor. *In general, any two full siblings have about one chance in four of sharing the same HLA type.* A sibling donor can have sickle trait but not sickle cell disease.

Because of the difficulty of finding an HLA-compatible donor without sickle cell disease among one's own siblings, sometimes another family member, or an unrelated person who is HLA compatible, can donate bone marrow instead. This procedure would be riskier than using a matched sibling donor and it is currently being studied in clinical research protocols at a number of transplant centers.

Haploidentical matches—those in which the donor is not a complete match for the recipient—are being performed in research settings. In cases like these, parents can be donors for their children, though complications such as graft rejection and graft-versus-host disease are more common. There are also studies testing reduced-intensity conditioning—in which the patient receives a lower dose of chemotherapy to prepare the body for the transplant—to possibly decrease long-term complications such as infertility, cancer, leukemia, and other serious problems. All of these alternative studies are in progress, and their safety and effectiveness are being determined at this time. Those interested in being considered for bone marrow transplant should talk to their physicians about being referred to a center participating in these studies for the latest information and discussion of their best options (see below).

The National Marrow Donor Program (NMDP) has been developed to assist in the search for compatible unrelated donors in the United States. Unfortunately, there are relatively few African-American donors in the registry, making it difficult for African-American patients in need of a transplant to find a donor. For more information, contact the NMDP at 1-800-MARROW2 or *www.bethematch.org*.

ELVIS'S STORY

Elvis Silva Magalhaes, at age 38, received a bone marrow transplant from his HLA-matched brother in Brasilia, Brazil. This made him one of the oldest people with sickle cell to have a BMT.

Elvis decided to have the bone marrow transplant after living for years with frequent pain, recurrent priapism, and leg ulcers. He recalls many sleepless nights because of sickle cell pain.

Today he is 52 years old and doing well, nearly fifteen years after his bone marrow transplant. He says that he didn't know how good it could feel to live without sickle cell pain. His only medication is daily penicillin because of his poor spleen function. He is among the leaders of ABRADFAL, the Brazilian advocacy group for sickle cell disease. Elvis is an international advocate for sickle cell patients, speaking and writing on their behalf to advocate for better services and treatments.

Recent studies at the NIH and other centers show that adults with sickle cell can undergo successful transplantation. Preparation for the transplant is different than for children, with less bone marrow destruction needed to house the donor cells.

QUALIFYING FOR A TRANSPLANTATION

Bone marrow transplants are not undertaken lightly. In order to qualify for one, the patient, doctor, and family must do a great deal of preparation:

1. *Sickle cell eligibility.* Start by talking with your child's or your sickle hema-

tologist. Whether the transplantation is appropriate to consider depends on whether the sickle cell disease is severe enough to justify the risks of bone marrow transplant.

Important points to consider are whether there have been stroke and chronic transfusion, frequent hospital stays for pain or lung problems, or other major sickle cell problems.

2. *Other medical issues.* Make your doctor aware that your family is considering the bone marrow transplant option. The BMT doctor needs to know as much as possible about your child, including all medical problems and whether they are related to sickle cell.

3. *HLA-typing blood tests.* HLA typing should be done on you or your child and the relative(s) with the highest probability of matching. Brothers or sisters from the same parents are the best potential donors as long as they do not have sickle cell disease. HLA typing may be costly. Parents and half-siblings are unlikely to match unless there's an unusual family tree. If the sibling is not a full HLA match, then alternate donor transplant may be considered as part of a clinical research trial.

4. *Psychosocial assessment.* The patient and family's ability to cope with the challenges of a BMT is just as important as medical information and typing. BMT is a complex and demanding process, and a family unlikely to go through it successfully may be better off choosing other treatment options. Factors such as adherence (making appointments and taking medications), support systems, comprehension, and finances all play a role in the psychosocial assessment. A parent or adult family member must be available to stay with the patient in the hospital during the month-long in-patient portion. Once discharged, the patient must expect to stay near the hospital (within about a 30-minute drive) for several months and come to the BMT clinic several times per week.

The cost of BMT may be more than $300,000, and insurance may not cover all costs. The patient must be prepared to take as many as five to ten medications daily. All of these factors combined make transplant a challenging process. The BMT social worker, financial counselor, and other members of the patient and family support team will help with the assessment and with making plans for a successful transplant.

5. *Pre-BMT evaluation.* After all of the above steps are completed and deci-

sions are made, scheduling the transplant can begin, which will be arranged by the BMT coordinator. A pre-BMT evaluation will be done over several visits. This includes medical testing of all the child's organs, blood tests and physical exams for both donor and recipient, and ongoing meetings with the BMT doctor to provide information and obtain informed consent. You should continue to ask all the questions you have. It is helpful to keep a notebook handy to jot down questions that come to mind.

THE TRANSPLANTATION PROCESS

Bone marrow transplantation can be described by dividing the process into three phases:

- preparation for transplantation (preparative regimen)
- transplantation
- post-transplantation management

Preparation for Transplantation (Preparative Regimen)

A central venous line (a large IV) will be inserted in the chest; it can remain in place for weeks or months. This is so that the patient does not have to get pricked for IVs and blood draws. Before transplantation, chemotherapy and drugs that suppress the immune system are given to the recipient.

Chemotherapy drugs, like those used in cancer patients, are used to destroy the recipient's bone marrow and immune system. This removes the sickle bone marrow, makes room for the donor's bone marrow to grow, and prevents the new donor marrow from being rejected. Chemotherapy drugs have many side effects. They are toxic to other organs in addition to the bone marrow. The BMT doctor will explain the short and long-term side effects of the specific drugs chosen for your child's transplant.

Some transplant techniques are using other ways to suppress the immune system besides chemotherapy. They kill immune system cells called lymphocytes by applying radiation to the lymph nodes. Medicines that are used in kidney transplant or heart transplant, such as sirolimus and anti-lymphocyte antibodies, are now also being used in some sickle cell transplants.

Transplantation

For a bone marrow transplant, donor bone marrow is usually taken from the large pelvic bones (back of the hips). The donor bone marrow is sucked out (doctors call this *aspiration*) with a special needle and syringe under general anesthesia, while the donor is asleep. The bone marrow is then given to the recipient intravenously through the central line.

Stem cells can also be removed from the donor's blood stream using an apheresis machine. The machine removes a part of the blood that contains the stem cells and returns the rest to the donor. This takes a number of hours, but is safer for the donor. Recent studies show that this way of collecting stem cells may not be as good for the recipient.

The bone marrow stem cells (the immature cells that will develop into the mature blood cell types) pass through the recipient's blood stream and find their way to the bone marrow cavities, where they will grow and mature if all goes well. Generally, two to four weeks are needed following transplantation before the transplanted marrow can produce enough mature red and white blood cells and platelets to sustain a healthy system.

Post-Transplantation Management
During the weeks following transplantation, there is no production of blood cells by the bone marrow in the recipient. Patients need to be isolated to protect against infection that can be life-threatening. Both bacterial and fungal infections can occur, but the infections can be treated with antibiotic and anti-fungal drugs. Painful mouth sores often develop, and intravenous narcotics are used to control pain. Platelet transfusions are necessary during this period to prevent serious bleeding. Packed red blood cells are transfused as needed until the new bone marrow can make enough red blood cells. If the donor and recipient are of different blood types, the blood type will change in the coming weeks.

Transplants done with immune suppression instead of chemotherapy could reduce the occurrence of these side effects of chemotherapy.

Nourishment
Chemotherapy often causes decreased appetite, nausea, and/or vomiting, which may make eating and drinking uncomfortable or even painful. These treatments may also interfere with stomach function and with the intestinal absorption of nutrients. Patients routinely require intravenous feeding. While intravenous feeding, or total parenteral nutrition (TPN), helps the host resist and overcome infections, it can also serve as an entryway for infections into the body. Scrupulous attention to caring for the intravenous feeding catheter and what enters it is therefore necessary.

Successful Transplantation

The average time needed for successful bone marrow transplantation is six to twelve months, including preparation, the transplant, recovery, and intensive follow-up. Doctors determine the success of the transplant by blood and genetic tests. They will look at the hemoglobin electrophoresis to see how much sickle hemoglobin is left. A test called a chimerism will show how much of the blood is from the donor at any given time.

COMPLICATIONS

Complications may follow even otherwise successful bone marrow transplantation. Such complications include:

- graft failure (the new bone marrow does not "take")
- infection
- graft-versus-host disease (GVHD), in which the donor cells attack the recipient's tissues
- cardiomyopathy (a disorder of the heart muscle)
- veno-occlusive disease of the liver (blockage of liver veins causing swelling, fluid retention, and jaundice, which may be life-threatening)
- pneumonia or other lung disease
- strokes, seizures, or bleeding in the brain
- high blood pressure
- kidney damage
- infertility (inability to produce children)
- hormone dysfunction (early menopause, low testosterone, thyroid problems)
- increased risk of developing cancer later in life

BMTs may also lead to cataracts (a clouding of the lens of the eye resulting in visual impairment). These are mostly the result of using steroids, such as prednisone, as part of the anti-rejection "cocktail." Steroids may also cause low potassium, bone loss, high blood sugar, mood and personality changes, kidney stones, and muscle wasting.

Graft Rejection/Failure

Graft failure happens when the donor's cells do not successfully grow in the recipient's body and the recipient's bone marrow will grow back, which means they will still have sickle cell disease. It is also possible that the bone

> **Features of the Chronic Form of GVHD**
> - Skin rashes
> - Inflammation of the corneas and conjunctivae (the outer lining of the corneas and the inner lining of the eyelids)
> - Inflammation of the mucous membranes of the mouth
> - Narrowing of the esophagus and inflammation of the intestines
> - Respiratory (lung) failure
> - Chronic liver damage
> - Wasting (loss of muscle, fat, and bone tissue)

marrow may not recover fast enough to fight life-threatening bleeding or infection, and death can occur. Graft failure may happen in up to 15% of matched sibling donor transplants for sickle cell disease.

Acute Graft-Versus-Host-Disease
Acute graft-versus-host disease (GVHD) happens when transplanted white blood cells fight against the recipient's tissues (the host). Even when the donor and the host are completely matched, there are usually minor differences between their cells.

Acute GVHD usually involves the skin, the digestive system, and the liver. A skin rash is often the first sign. Diarrhea, abdominal pain, and intestinal paralysis may result from the intestinal involvement. Liver dysfunction may also occur. Severe immunologic deficiency may develop with a risk of life-threatening infection and death.

Chronic graft-versus-host disease may develop later and last much longer. GVHD can usually be prevented or controlled with powerful immune-suppressing drugs, although these carry dangers of their own. It is essential that the recipient take the daily medication to prevent GVHD. Because GVHD can be debilitating and life-threatening, it is one of the main reasons that BMT is not offered to more sickle cell patients; it is possible that GVHD may be as bad as, or even worse than, having sickle cell disease itself.

Infertility

Transplantation of bone marrow or cord blood stem cells can cure sickle cell disease, but many of the treatments that prepare the body to accept the transplanted cells have a side effect of infertility for males and females. Newer experimental transplant preparative treatments using less chemotherapy may have lower risk of infertility. Males can try sperm banking before the transplant, but the sperm may also have low function due to sickle cell. It is important to remember that even after transplantation the patient's sperm or eggs will still carry the genes for sickle cell disease, not the genes of the marrow donor.

You are still at risk for having a child with sickle cell disease (See Chapter 7). Discuss the risks of infertility when you meet with transplant doctors.

THE FUTURE OF BONE MARROW TRANSPLANTATION

Research is now under way to expand the option of BMT to more patients and to reduce the high risk of complications. One approach is called *reduced intensity transplant*. This uses lower doses of chemotherapy in combination with powerful immune-suppressing drugs and sometimes low doses of radiation therapy. This approach appears to make transplant safer and easier for adults with sickle cell, which means more patients could be cured.

Other efforts focus on using alternate donors in patients who do not have fully matched siblings available. The alternate-donor source may be from cord blood, an incompletely matched relative, or an unrelated volunteer donor. The proportion of African-American donors must be increased to make this approach successful, and the NMDP has efforts under way to increase minority representation. Invite the NMDP campaign called "Be The Match" to your community to recruit more marrow donors.

15

Gene Therapy for Sickle Cell Disease

Effective treatment for sickle cell disease has developed slowly over the last fifty years, to the frustration of both doctors treating sickle cell and individuals living with the disease. But recent research progress has shown that gene therapy could be a promising treatment and possible cure.

In general terms, sickle cell disease can be cured using bone marrow transplantation (see Chapter 14) or gene therapy. Bone marrow transplant is already being used for sickle cell patients who have found a donor with compatible bone marrow. However, gene therapy offers hope for a universal cure that can be offered to everyone without needing to find a donor match—all that is needed is the patient's own cells.

GENE THERAPY TERMS

Bone Marrow Stem Cells

Human bone marrow contains special cells known as adult stem cells, which are needed to make all types of blood cells in the body—red cells, white cells, and platelets. Following a bone marrow transplant, these adult stem cells from the donor help correct the patient's sickle cell mutation, allowing the patient's body to create its own normal red blood cells. Bone marrow adult stem cells are different from embryonic stem cells that come from human embryos; the two types should not be confused.

Genetic Code

To understand gene therapy research, it helps to know about the genetic code. DNA contains the genetic code, or instructions, used to make proteins in living cells. Changes to the genetic code are also responsible for mutations that cause human disease. A mutation in a person's DNA can

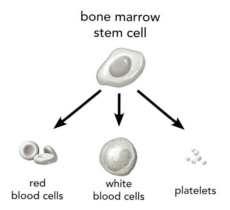

change the way the body produces certain proteins such as hemoglobin S, the protein in red blood cells that allows blood to carry oxygen throughout the body. One goal of gene therapy is to correct DNA mutations, allowing the patient's body to produce proteins correctly and essentially curing the patient's condition.

Sickle Beta Gene

In this chapter we'll be focusing on the sickle beta gene, which is a mutation that causes the body to produce abnormal hemoglobin. This abnormal hemoglobin causes red blood cells to sickle, which leads to the complications we see in sickle cell disease. Through gene therapy, researchers are attempting to either repair the sickle beta gene or replace it with a normal gene in order to cure sickle cell disease.

WHAT IS GENE THERAPY?

Gene therapy is an emerging treatment utilizing the addition of properly-functioning genes or the repair of mutated genes to treat genetic diseases such as sickle cell disease. Diseases like sickle cell that are caused by a single mutation have been a logical first choice for gene therapy treatment. Researchers are experimenting with ways to cure sickle cell disease by correcting the sickle beta gene or inserting a normal beta hemoglobin gene into bone marrow stem cells from sickle cell patients.

Types of Gene Therapy

There are two major types of gene therapy. Germ line gene therapy involves the correction or addition of normal genes to germ cells (sperm or eggs). This change would then be passed on to later generations. This approach may cure genetic diseases, but it is not currently permitted in humans, not only because of technical limitations but also a question of whether it is an ethical practice.

The second type is somatic gene therapy, in which normal genes are added to somatic cells (cells in the body that are not germ cells). Any change in DNA will only occur in the person receiving treatment, and the change will not be inherited by later generations. Somatic gene therapy is the method used to develop gene therapy treatments for sickle cell disease.

Gene Therapy Methods
There are different ways to design gene therapy to treat human disease. The most common method is to add a new gene at a random location within the patient's DNA to allow the patient's body to create normal proteins. Other methods include replacing the mutated gene with a normal gene or repairing the gene mutation, both of which have been accomplished but are very difficult to do.

HOW WILL GENE THERAPY BE DONE FOR SICKLE CELL DISEASE?

The most widely researched gene therapy method for treating sickle cell uses viruses. A virus can attach itself to cells and places its genetic material inside the cells as a means of survival. From there, the infected cells grow and cause disease. Taking advantage of this natural process, researchers have developed viruses called viral vectors that carry normal genes into human cells. To accomplish this, the virus's disease-causing genes are removed and replaced with a normal human gene. Once inside the body, instead of spreading disease the viral vector inserts the normal gene into the DNA of the body's cells.

In March 2017, the *New England Journal of Medicine* published "Gene Therapy in a Patient with Sickle Cell Disease," a report of the first successful case of using gene therapy in a patient with sickle cell disease. In this case, a fifteen-year-old boy in Paris, France, received an antisickling variant of hemoglobin through a stem cell transplant, and two years later he had been cured of all the symptoms of severe sickle cell disease. This is the first reported gene therapy cure.

Other ways to produce a gene therapy cure for sickle cell disease are still being studied. Gene editing with a technique called CRISPR has been making rapid progress since 2015, though it has not yet been studied in human sickle cell disease as of August 2018. Non-viral vectors such as bacteria

DNA, fat droplets, DNA by itself, or any combination of these have also been used to add genes to cells, but their success has been limited. The focus in this chapter will be on the exciting progress made toward gene therapy using viral vectors.

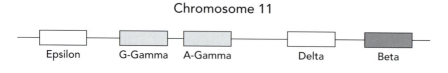

Hemoglobin genes on chromosome 11

GENE THERAPY OFFERS THE PROMISE OF A CURE FOR ALL

Since the early 1980s, researchers have been working on gene therapy for sickle cell disease, pursuing two main approaches. Some are investigating whether repairing the sickle beta gene or adding a normal gene into adult stem cells will produce a cure. Another special approach involves turning off the sickle beta gene and turning on the fetal gamma gene, which produces the type of hemoglobin found in babies before they are born. This hemoglobin is better at transporting oxygen than the hemoglobin produced by the sickle beta gene. Progress is being made, and there is a real possibility of a cure—but some technical challenges still have to be overcome.

A major breakthrough in gene therapy for sickle cell happened in 2002, when researchers from Harvard University cured sickle cell disease in a mouse by using a lentivirus vector. Researchers removed bone marrow containing the sickle beta gene from the mouse and genetically "corrected" it by the addition of a normal beta gene. The corrected stem cells were transplanted into other mice with sickle cell to produce a cure. A similar process exists in which a patient's own stem cells are removed, genetically corrected, and given back to the same patient—a process known as autologous stem cell transplant.

An improved version of the lentivirus vector, developed to be safer for humans and causing fewer side effects, has recently been used to treat sickle cell disease. The researchers at Harvard, working with a group of French researchers, have redesigned the viral vector with a modified normal human beta gene. They treated beta thalassemia first, with positive results. The researchers moved on to treat a patient with sickle cell disease with this method and achieved a cure; this is the case noted in the March 2017 *New England Journal of Medicine* article.

Since that time, more children with severe combined immune deficiency have been treated safely in many countries around the world and cured with the new viral vector. More importantly, they have not developed leukemia. The same viral vector will be used to treat sickle cell disease. The researchers at Harvard, working with the French group, have redesigned the viral vector with a modified normal human beta gene. They treated beta thalassemia first. If successful, then the same vector will be used to treat stem cell from patients with sickle cell. The research community is eagerly awaiting the results of these important studies.

Another group of scientists at St. Jude Children's Research Hospital, using the lentivirus vector, joined parts of the fetal gamma and sickle beta genes together to cure sickle cell disease in mice. The gamma gene produces fetal hemoglobin, which blocks the problems caused by sickle beta hemoglobin. This design may work well in sickle cell patients, but studies so far have found that this method does not produce enough fetal hemoglobin. More research is ongoing.

In the past, it had been a challenge to collect a sufficient amount of stem cells from bone marrow or blood for gene therapy. In 2007, a group at the Whitehead Institute for Biomedical Research addressed this problem by developing a method to take skin cells (fibroblasts) and treat them in the laboratory with growth factors to produce a new source of stem cells. These cells are called induced pluripotent stem (iPS) cells. This new research was developed to cure sickle cell disease in mice, providing the first direct proof that skin cells can be used to treat a genetic disease. Subsequent research has shown that iPS cells can also be generated from cells in blood and urine. More work is still needed before iPS cells can be used for human disease.

HOW THE FIRST GENE THERAPY WAS FIRST GIVEN

The first application of gene therapy for sickle cell was done with autologous stem cell transplant. In this procedure, some of the patient's own bone marrow cells were removed, then the stem cells were isolated and genetically corrected. The patient's remaining marrow was partially destroyed using drugs to "make room" for the genetically changed stem cells, which were then returned to the patient. Autologous transplant carries fewer serious risks than a bone marrow transplant using a donor with matching marrow, the method currently used to cure sickle cell disease, because the patient is receiving his or her own stem cells. This means the patient can avoid the

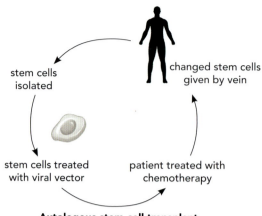

Autologous stem cell transplant

complications that occur when the immune system reacts to new cells that come from another person. More research is needed to determine the best way to achieve safe autologous stem cell transplant.

Umbilical cord blood also contains stem cells that can be used for gene therapy. Parents can choose to donate their newborn's cord blood to a public storage bank at no cost or store it in a private bank for a fee. Read more about cord blood banking at https://parentsguidecordblood.org/en.

BARRIERS TO SUCCESSFUL GENE THERAPY

We still have a long way to go before consistently successful gene therapy is achieved. These are just some of the challenges researchers still face:

- The new gene may not continue to consistently produce protein. To be considered a true cure, there would not be a need to repeat the therapy.

- Any time a foreign material—even a single gene—is put into human cells, that material will be attacked by the body's immune system.

- Viruses are the delivery method of choice in most gene therapy studies, but they may produce unwanted side effects by interfering with other genes in the patient's DNA.

- There is always the fear that once inside the patient, the viral vector may recover its ability to cause disease, despite efforts to prevent this.

- If the viral vector inserts the DNA in the wrong location, it could cause cancer.

Ethical and legal issues are also of great concern when discussing gene therapy. A review board known as the Recombinant Advisory Committee

(RAC) was developed to address these concerns. Gene therapy could wipe out genetic diseases before they begin and eliminate human suffering; it has tremendous potential for the future.

However, there are many ethical concerns. First, it puts human fate in our own hands, giving scientists the ability to manufacture people. Some are concerned that gene therapy will be used to create a superior race. But the idea of gene therapy is to cure hereditary diseases, not to make any race superior. Another consideration is religion. Some consider it sinful to manipulate DNA. But somatic stem cell gene therapy is not passed to offspring; it allows the next generation to make its own decisions about medical treatment.

Some people feel that gene therapy may be difficult to regulate, and it could become available on the black market. It could be used for any genetically linked trait such as appearance or physical enhancement.

Lastly, invasion of privacy is always a concern for many. Insurance companies could make it mandatory for customers to have genetic screening before they are issued a policy. This could cause discrimination against families with genetic diseases.

FUTURE OUTLOOK

Gene therapy has been progressing slowly, but it has the potential to successfully treat cancer, cystic fibrosis, diabetes, Parkinson's disease, and certain kinds of heart disease. Gene therapy has been largely ineffective and controversial, but it is the most promising approach to curing genetic diseases. Like every other new medical advance, it will take time to develop.

In late 2018, the NIH announced the "Cure Sickle Cell Initiative." This ambitious plan aims to take the latest genetic discoveries and technological advances to safely move promising genetic-based curative therapies into clinical trials for sickle cell within five to ten years.

Although much work remains, the future promises better and safer gene therapy tools and, eventually, a cure. One study has reported success in snipping out the DNA in a stem cell that contains the sickle mutation and inserting the normal DNA sequence, effectively curing sickle cell disease with efficiency and accuracy. These modified stem cells are able to create normal hemoglobin in a laboratory to a level of about 20%. This study also shows that these cells are able to be transplanted successfully into immune-deficient mice, although the mice don't go on to produce as much normal hemoglobin as in lab settings.

While there are still obstacles ahead, it appears that gene therapy offers promise as a true cure for sickle cell disease. Perhaps in the near future our goal of making sickle cell the first molecular disease cured in all individuals will be realized because of the great advances we are achieving in molecular genetic research.

16

Participating in Sickle Cell Research

Even as you read this, people around the world are working to find new medications and treatments for sickle cell disease. This research starts in laboratory and animal studies and goes on in the form of *clinical trials*, in which new medications and methods are tested both for their effectiveness and their safety in individuals with sickle cell disease. Sickle cell patients and families should consider helping find new treatments that will improve many lives, including their own. Without patients willing to participate, there will be no new advances in sickle cell treatment. No new drugs are approved for use by the FDA without extensive clinical trials showing safety and effectiveness.

Patients who take part in such studies often do better than patients who do not, because the study provides expert medical care, the latest information, free lab studies, and free treatment. To find the latest research in a particular area, go to the website *www.ClinicalTrials.gov* and search the phrase "sickle cell." You may also contact your nearest medical school or university, or your primary care provider, to learn about research going on in your area.

PLACEBO CONTROLS

Some trials will be designed to compare the treatment to an inactive treatment call a placebo. A placebo is an inactive pill, liquid, or powder that looks like the real medication, but has no treatment value. In such trials, some patients will be given the active medication being explored, but others will be given a placebo. The other way to see if new treatments are effective is to have a "control" group that gets the standard treatment.

AN INTRODUCTION TO CLINICAL TRIALS

Choosing to participate in a clinical trial is an important personal decision that most people don't want to make alone. Instead, they talk to their physician and to family members or friends before deciding. Once you have identified trials that might help you, contact the study research staff and ask questions about these trials. That way, you'll know that the decision you make will be a good one. Next, you should review the protocol for the clinical trial.

What Is a Protocol?

A protocol is a study plan on which all clinical trials are based. The plan is carefully designed to safeguard the health of the participants as well as to answer specific research questions. A protocol describes what types of people may participate in the trial; the schedule of tests, procedures, medications, and dosages; and the length of the study. While they are in a clinical trial, participants following a protocol are seen regularly by the research staff for the purpose of monitoring their health and determining the safety and effectiveness of their treatment.

Treatment trials test new treatments, new combinations of drugs, or new approaches to surgery or radiation therapy.

Clinical Trials: Benefits and Risks

The benefits of participating in clinical trials are that you:

- play an active role in your health care;
- gain access to new research treatments before they are widely available;
- obtain expert medical care at leading healthcare facilities during the trial; and
- help others by contributing to medical research.

The risks involved in clinical trials include:

- possible unpleasant, serious, or even life-threatening side effects to treatment; and
- the chance that you will not receive the active treatment or that the treatment may not work for you

Prevention trials look for better ways to prevent disease in people, or for ways to prevent a disease from returning. These approaches may include medicines, vitamins, vaccines, minerals, or lifestyle changes.

Screening trials test the best way to detect diseases or health conditions.

Quality of life trials (or *supportive care trials*) explore ways to improve the comfort and quality of life of people who must live with a chronic illness.

What Are the Phases of Clinical Trials?

Clinical trials are conducted in phases. The trials at each phase have a different purpose and help scientists answer different questions:

- In *Phase I trials*, researchers test, for the first time, a new drug or treatment in a small group of people (20 to 80) to evaluate its safety, determine a safe dosage range, and identify side effects.
- In *Phase II trials*, the drug or treatment is given to a larger group of people (dozens or hundreds) in order to find out more about its safety and effectiveness.
- In *Phase III trials*, the study drug or treatment is given to large groups of people (hundreds or thousands) to confirm its effectiveness, monitor side effects, compare it to commonly used treatments, and collect information that will allow the drug or treatment to be used safely.
- In *Phase IV trials*, drugs or treatments already approved by the Food and Drug Administration are studied to find additional information, including risks, benefits, and optimal use.

PINPOINT, an upcoming tablet and smartphone app for teens with SCD, is an example of a quality of life trial in which two of the authors of this book are currently involved. PINPOINT improves self-care for teens by providing information about SCD including causes, treatments, and self-care options. A great benefit of PINPOINT is the fact that it makes it easier for parents and healthcare teams to get information from adolescent SCD patients because it utilizes a tech medium that teens are comfortable with and enjoy. Acquiring pain data and other information through this app allows healthcare teams and family members to adjust and improve treatment plans.

What Happens During a Clinical Trial?

The trial team includes doctors and nurses as well as social workers and other healthcare professionals. They check the health of the participant at the beginning of the trial, give specific instructions for participating in the trial, monitor the participant carefully during the trial, and stay in touch after the trial is completed.

Some clinical trials involve more tests and doctor visits than the participant would normally have for an illness or condition. For all types of trials, the participant works with a research team. Frequent contact with research staff members yields the best likelihood of getting a correct answer for the trial.

What Is Informed Consent?

Informed consent means that you are given and understand all the information you need to make an informed decision about whether or not you want to participate in a research study.. It is also means that you will be given further information during each stage of the trial. To help you decide whether or not to participate, the doctors and nurses involved in the trial explain it in detail. If your native language isn't English, a translator can be provided. It is the researcher's responsibility to explain it in a way that you understand. If you have questions, you should ask them before agreeing to participate. Make sure you understand what you are being asked to do and what the risks and benefits will be. Once you have understood the explanation, you'll be given an informed consent document that includes details about the study, such as, its purpose, duration, required procedures, and key contacts. Risks and potential benefits are also explained in the document. Then the researcher of staff member will ask if you're ready to decide whether or not to sign the document. Informed consent is not a contract, and the participant may withdraw from the trial at any time.

What Are Some of the Key Issues You Should Discuss with the Research Team?

The team will want you to know as much as possible about the clinical trial and feel comfortable asking questions. You'll want to know what care you'll be provided while the trial goes on, and what part, if any, of the trial treatment you will have to pay for.

The following are the kinds of questions you'll want answers to. All of the answers to these questions should be found in the informed consent document.

- What is the purpose of the study?
- Who is going to be in the study?
- Why do researchers believe the new treatment being tested may be effective? Has it been tested before?
- What kinds of tests and treatments are involved?
- How do the possible risks, side effects, and benefits in the study compare with those of my current treatment?
- How might this trial affect my daily life?
- How long will the trial last?
- Will hospitalization be required?
- Who will pay for the treatment?
- What will I or my insurance have to pay?
- Will I be reimbursed for other expenses?
- What type of long-term follow-up care is part of this study?
- How will I know that the treatment is working?
- Will results of the trials be provided to me?
- Who will be in charge of my care?

The protocol may require more of your time and attention than you can give when first asked to participate. Take it home and share it with your family to help with your decision. If you are not sure about participating, it is better not to start the study.

How Safe is the Trial?

The ethical and legal codes that govern medical practice in general also apply to clinical trials. Most clinical research is federally regulated and monitored, with built-in safeguards to protect you throughout the course of the trial. The trial follows a carefully controlled protocol.

Your protection doesn't stop there. While the trial is going on, your team will report results at scientific meetings, publish interim findings in medical journals, and also report interim findings to various government agencies.

In addition, every clinical trial in the United States must be approved and monitored by an institutional review board (IRB) to make sure the risks are as low as possible, as measured against the disease itself. An IRB is an independent committee of physicians, statisticians, community advocates, and others who work to ensure that a clinical trial is ethical and that the rights of study participants are protected. By federal regulation, all institutions that conduct or support biomedical research involving humans must have an IRB that initially approves and periodically reviews the research.

If there is an intervention, there will be an independent group of experts reviewing the recruitment of subjects, adverse results, and data to make sure it is safe and will answer the research questions. This is called a Data Safety Monitoring Board. The study will be stopped when it answers the research question, if it will not get an answer, or it is found to not be safe.

In a Nutshell

People, and especially minorities, sometimes avoid clinical trials because they fear they will be "experimented on." In fact, doctors and clinics that conduct clinical trials are usually the best in their field, and can offer you the best possible care with the latest treatment. Participating in a trial will lower your costs and provide you with services you might otherwise not have been able to get. The most important reason to participate is that you may help make new treatments available that may benefit you and many other individuals with sickle cell disease. Check out the facts about clinical trials that could help you make an informed decision.

17

What You Can Do

THE POWER OF ONE

In 1984, in Atlanta, when her son Carey was eight, doctors told Berrutha Harper that her son would die of sickle cell disease before he reached his teen years. Berrutha had to take her son to the local emergency rooms for pain treatment, and she often experienced long waits and had to deal with healthcare providers who had little or no sickle cell experience.

When Berrutha saw that she couldn't get consistently good care in ordinary emergency rooms, she began to dream of an emergency room dedicated to the needs of sickle cell patients, with a specially trained staff of healthcare providers who would treat patients with knowledge and compassion.

Berrutha was the kind of dreamer who saw a dream as possibility. She organized other parents and patients into a group of people who could share concerns about sickle cell patients and consider how to improve sickle cell care in the largest of the Atlanta hospitals, Grady Memorial.

The hospital received many patient complaints each day about the care given to emergency room sickle cell patients. But the hospital's official position was that it couldn't afford an emergency room dedicated exclusively to the treatment of sickle cell patients.

Berrutha was not the kind of woman to give up easily. She set out to get state funding from the legislature. During lunch breaks from her job as a medical clerk in a local healthcare clinic, she would go to the state capitol building and knock on legislators' doors.

One day, a patient came into the emergency room with chest pain, and was treated for sickle cell pain crisis. The patient died of a heart attack, a diagnosis not thought of because the patient had sickle cell disease. Berrutha called all of the parent/patient groups to stage a protest march in front of the state capitol. Berrutha arrived at the capitol with signs in hand, but no people showed up to march. A discouraged Berrutha sat on the steps and sent up a short prayer. A group of school bus drivers from South Georgia, who had delivered school children for a capitol tour, asked Berrutha about the protest signs and got an education about sickle cell disease. The bus drivers asked if they could carry the signs for Berrutha, as they would be there waiting for the school kids to return. The news of the marching bus drivers reached the inner chambers of the legislators in session. The leader of the Black Caucus came outside and invited Berrutha to meet with him if she would call off the march. This was the first time Berrutha's story was heard by the influential leaders of the legislature. Funds were allocated to Grady Memorial Hospital to start a 24-hour clinic with a dedicated staff of healthcare providers trained to care for sickle cell patients.

In September 1984, the Sickle Cell Center opened its doors for patients. It has been open ever since, providing round-the-clock emergency care, comprehensive preventive care, research, in-patient consultations, and education. All of this was the result of one mother's prayer, vision, and perseverance.

FUNDRAISING

There are several ways to raise money for your sickle cell activities. First, set up or partner with a 501(c)(3) tax-exempt organization so donations can be tax deductible. Many hospitals, churches, and civic groups have this status. Plan a budget. Funds will be needed for scholarships for college, emergency needs of patients, research projects, and education. Fundraising activities include walk-a-thons, bowl-a-thons, banquets, and concerts. Invite corporate participation, and invite the local press to do a story on the event. This will raise awareness about sickle cell disease and raise funds at the same time.

COMMUNITY-BASED SICKLE CELL PROGRAMS

There are many community-based sickle programs throughout the country that provide counseling, education, and many direct services to patients and their families. They promote funding and services for sickle cell. They also have therapy groups, summer camps for children, and vocational support programs. Become a volunteer to help them improve the lives of individuals with sickle cell disease and their families.

PEER MENTORING

Peer mentoring in transition clinics and camps is an important activity that requires participation from individuals with sickle cell disease. They are the authorities on living with sickle cell disease and have credibility with the youth learning how to best manage their lives and disease. Not only do the youth benefit from their wisdom, but our older patients serving as mentors have really enjoyed the activities and felt a real and appropriate sense of pride in what they were doing.

BLOOD DRIVES

It is important to reduce the formation of antibodies in sickle cell patients. The best way to do this is to transfuse blood from people of the same ethnic background. If sickle cell disease primarily affects those in the African-American community in your area, then blood donations should be increased in that community to reduce the antigen exposure. The more antibodies a patient makes, the more difficult it is to find blood that matches and will not cause a transfusion reaction.

Get involved by organizing a blood drive in your office, civic group, or church group. Contact the American Red Cross or other local blood donation centers that can help you set up a blood drive. Ask about a directed donation program, in which a group of donors can be matched to a specific sickle cell patient to reduce the blood exposure and reduce the making of antibodies. At the blood drives, educate the public about sickle cell disease and the need for regular blood donations.

BONE MARROW DONOR REGISTRY

The National Marrow Donor Program at *www.bethematch.org* helps organize testing for potential bone marrow donors. As transplants increase as options for sickle cell patients, a larger list of potential donors will increase the success of finding a match. This program is great to offer while doing blood drives and helps raise awareness of sickle cell disease.

HEALTH FAIRS

Health fairs are good places to educate the public about sickle cell disease. Set up a table with informational handouts, and have people on hand to answer questions. If possible, provide sickle cell screenings by drawing blood for hemoglobin electrophoresis. You can network with other community-based health organizations to help support sickle cell patients.

PUBLIC EDUCATION

Educate the public in your community by inviting the local newspaper and TV news to do stories about patients and events in your area. Sickle cell patients have wonderfully inspirational life stories of overcoming pain and hardship. Talk about innovative support groups or new advances in research.

POLITICS

Get out the vote for individuals who will support issues important to those with sickle cell disease and their families. Tell your legislators about sickle cell disease and the need for services in your community. States can be involved in newborn screening, funding comprehensive centers, funding vocational rehabilitation programs, and funding preventive care. You can contact legislators by newsletters, personal calls, personal visits, and e-mail. Invite them to your educational events. National leaders need to be educated about the unique needs of sickle cell patients and the need for increased research funding. Sickle cell is the most common genetic disease in the United States, but it is underfunded compared to other, less common genetic diseases such as hemophilia and cystic fibrosis.

Make the Most of Your Meeting with Legislators or Their Staff

You have an appointment with a legislator, executive, or legislative aide—congratulations! You will probably have a limited time, only 15 to 30 minutes, so you want to be prepared to make the most of this time! Here are suggestions to help you have a successful meeting.

Coordinate your advocacy efforts with others—it will be a stronger message for action if many groups of people unify to advocate the same goals for sickle cell rather than if each person suggests a different goal.

Thank them for their support for Americans suffering from sickle cell disease. This is a good way to start off the meeting positively and will show them that you appreciate their efforts.

Prepare an outline of your message: the "talking points." If you are coming as a group, assign each person to speak about one point.

- Tell your story. Prepare personal stories and anecdotes to share.

→ Make the case for one or two goals. Give statistics from your community that illustrate why the current funding does not meet the need.

→ Ask for a commitment to support increased funding for sickle cell. Your goals are to enlist support for the next fiscal year's funding requests as well as the long-term support of sickle cell treatment and research programs. It is important to be as specific as you can.

Thank them for the meeting, and follow up promptly. Let them know that you appreciate their work and taking the time to meet with you. Send them any information or materials that you promised during the meeting.

If you meet with an aide or other staff member, be respectful and do not be discouraged. Legislators depend on their staffs to help them keep track of the numerous issues that are important to the communities they represent. Legislative aides are often very knowledgeable on your issues, and they have substantial influence over their legislator. Regardless of their title or age, they can help make policy decisions and can be very important allies in helping victims.

The same approach can be used for letters or other communication, even if it is not a face-to-face meeting.

Adapted from a Sickle Cell Disease Association of America handout.

SICKLE CELL CAMP

Many sickle cell centers and foundations in major cities have annual sickle cell summer camps for children. Camp is a way for children to interact with their peers in a fun environment. Older individuals with sickle cell disease are a source of knowledge and inspiration for younger children with the disease. Usually, medical support is provided by the medical teams from the sickle cell centers. Campers are encouraged to drink extra fluids, take rest breaks, and avoid high-temperature exposure. These camps typically charge a small fee to cover lodging and food. Frequently, scholarships are provided to those who do not have any resources. To locate a camp, contact the nearest sickle cell center or the Sickle Cell Disease Association of America for the chapter nearest to you.

WHY SUPPORT AND COUNSELING ARE VITAL

Sickle cell disease is not only an anemia of the blood. Like all serious illnesses it affects every aspect of the patient's life, and the physical ills can be made worse by intense emotional and social stress. Without proper medical attention and support from those organized to help, the psychological component of this disease can prove to be as devastating as the disease itself.

In some respects, better treatment and care of sickle cell patients have intensified the emotional and psychological problems associated with the disease. Because life expectancies have increased, patients can face a seemingly unending prospect of absence from school and work, poor employment prospects, and managed-care crises. Depression, boredom, and antisocial or self-destructive behaviors are expressions of the intense emotional strain the patient faces daily.

The very good news is that sickle cell patients don't have to face the disease alone. From initial screening through every stage and pain episode, counseling and support are available. One only has to look.

Not only is immediate help available to the patient, but counseling and support are also there for family, friends, teachers, employers, and healthcare professionals. In fact, the interconnected efforts of the entire sickle cell community are the key to successful support.

What we offer you here, to start you on your journey, is a basic list of the resources that will get you started. Once you take the first step, you'll find that the appropriate path will be obvious. Simply walk it, as you do any walk, one step at a time. What you will soon see is that each organization is a link in a long, interconnected chain of support, a chain that has grown much stronger in the past thirty years, as we have all come to better understand the needs of the sickle cell patient.

Once you start, you'll soon find that there are different kinds of support groups available:

- Some agencies are government-sponsored, but many are community-based.
- Some focus on education and clinical research for the medical community.

What You Can Do

- Some stress political activism in their efforts to generate the funds for clinical research and community-outreach programs.
- Others stress one-on-one personal involvement and individual care.

Whatever the approach, their goal is the same—to fight for the health and rights of the individual sickle cell patient.

A list of resources to help you on your way is found in the Resources section at the end of this book.

PART 4

SICKLE CELL TRAIT AND GENETICS

18

Sickle Cell Trait

INCIDENCE

Sickle cell trait occurs when a person inherits of just one sickle gene and one normal hemoglobin A gene. These individuals are also called sickle cell carriers. Just under half the hemoglobin inside the red blood cells is sickle hemoglobin. More than 3.5 million African Americans are carriers of sickle cell trait. Sickle cell trait is common in Central Africa, around the Mediterranean, and throughout the Middle, Near and Far East. This occurred because children with sickle trait are less likely to die when they are infected with malaria, a very common red blood cell parasite that infects almost every person in these areas. Up to 25% of young children with malaria infection die in the first years of life. Young children with sickle trait who become infected with malaria parasites do not get as sick and are less likely to die because the parasite cannot grow well in the red cell that contain half sickle hemoglobin and half normal hemoglobin.

Thalassemia and other hemoglobin disorders are also common in all parts of the world where malaria was common because they make malaria infection somewhat less severe. It is also common in the Caribbean, South America, and many other parts of the world where it was introduced by the slave trades and later migrations.

WHAT DOES SICKLE TRAIT MEAN TO ME?
Individuals with sickle cell trait do not have the disease and will not develop sickle cell disease in the future. However, they are at risk for having a child with sickle cell disease if their partner also has sickle cell trait. They may also have a child with sickle cell disease if their partner carries a gene for beta thalassemia or other hemoglobins that interact with sickle

hemoglobin like Hb C, D, E, O, and others. If you have already had a child with sickle cell disease, you and your partner are both carriers of Hb S or one of these other hemoglobin disorders.

You should be certain of your diagnosis, because some people have been told they have sickle cell trait when they really have a variant of the disease. If in doubt, have a complete blood count and hemoglobin electrophoresis test repeated and reviewed by hematologist who knows about hemoglobin disorders. Sickle cell trait is important to you because:

- You can pass this gene on to your future children.
- Sickle cell trait will never transform into sickle cell disease.
- You should have a normal life without symptoms.
- You may need to take some precautions if you plan to push yourself to the extremes of human endurance like climbing high mountains, exercising to extreme dehydration, and exercising after going from sea level to high altitude.

You or your children may have to be tested and report your carrier status before participating in National Collegiate Athletic Association athletic activities.

MISDIAGNOSIS

People with sickle cell trait are generally completely normal physically, show no symptoms, and have normal laboratory tests. Their complete blood count evaluation is normal with no anemia and no evidence of red cells breaking apart. There are no abnormalities other than hemoglobin AS on hemoglobin electrophoresis.

If symptoms more typical of sickle cell disease—like anemia, pains, and jaundice—occur, the following should be considered:

- Misdiagnosed sickle β^+ thalassemia. A person with sickle β^+ thalassemia may have symptoms of sickle cell disease. Always get tests and counsel from healthcare providers who understand the different types of sickle cell disease.
- Misdiagnosed sickle plus some other interacting hemoglobin like C, D, or E.
- Incorrect diagnosis. Individuals with hemoglobin SC disease are sometimes told that they have sickle trait by uninformed health professionals. This can be correctly diagnosed with a repeat he-

moglobin electrophoresis that is reviewed by an individual with knowledge of hemoglobin disorders.

SICKLE CELL TRAIT COMPLICATIONS

There are some uncommon complications that do occasionally occur in individuals with sickle cell trait. There may be blood in the urine that usually can't be seen without looking with a microscope. This occurs in 1%–4% of individuals with sickle trait. Blood that is visible without a microscope occurs very rarely. If you see blood in your urine, you should see a physician because causes other than sickle trait are more likely, such as kidney or bladder stones, polyps, tumors, or bleeding disorders. Extremely rarely, the bleeding lasts for an extended period and iron and other treatments may be needed. Drinking a lot of water and getting plenty of bed rest may stop these bleeding episodes if done quickly. Individuals with bleeding into the urine should drink a lot of water before, during, and after physical exertion. Those with frequent, severe, or persistent bleeding into the urine may need to avoid activities that regularly cause episodes.

Individuals with sickle trait may have a higher risk for blood clots in the legs that go to the lungs. No special prevention is need over that recommended for the general population. Management of blood clots, if they develop, is presently the same as the general population.

VERY RARE COMPLICATIONS

Complications such as splenic infarction, pain episodes, and sudden death may be caused by severe cases of hypoxia and dehydration or by overexertion, especially at high altitude. Fortunately, these complications are rare, and there are only sporadic case reports in the medical journals. There is no good predictor of which individuals with sickle cell trait will have these complications when placed under extreme conditions.

Individuals with sickle trait have a higher risk of serious complications if they exercise at the extremes of human endurance. This was recently publicized by the coaches of the National Collegiate Athletic Association after a few athletes died during rigorous football practice, some with sickle trait who died of heat/dehydration-related sickling and some without sickle trait who died of heatstroke. The intensity of exercise that causes problems in sickle cell trait also may cause problems, even death, in individuals who do not have sickle trait. The risk is higher, however, in those with sickle trait. The US military found a solution to this issue decades ago and modified military training to prevent deaths among military recruits. Not only did the occurrence of these deaths decrease in individuals with trait, but basic training was made safer for all recruits. The NCAA now requires all athletes at Division I and II schools to either be tested for the trait or decline testing before competing. Many have suggested it would be reasonable to follow the successful lead of the military and insist athletic coaches should modify training methods for all athletes to avoid medical complications from overexertion.

Extremely low oxygen levels, exercise at high altitude, and dehydration can cause painful damage to the spleen (splenic infarction). Interestingly, Caucasians with sickle cell trait may be at higher risk for these complications. Drinking a lot of water regularly and building up exercise tolerance are important preventive measures.

Splenic Syndrome

The symptoms of splenic syndrome are:

- abdominal pain, especially in the upper-left abdominal area, and left shoulder pain
- nausea, vomiting, fever, and jaundice
- enlargement of the spleen

This occurs at altitudes over 9,000 feet in individuals who reside at sea level and exercise vigorously shortly after arriving at that altitude. If you are concerned about splenic infarction, go to an emergency room and tell the medical staff that you have sickle cell trait. Splenic syndrome may not be a complication the staff is aware of if they do not see many sickle cell patients. Treatment is usually pain control, hydration, and supportive measures, at which point the episode usually resolves. Rarely, spleen removal may be required.

Multi-Organ Failure and Sudden Death

There have been case reports in military and sports medical journals of sudden collapse and death in individuals with sickle cell trait as a result of extreme physical activity and little hydration. In one military study of two million recruits, a 28-fold increase in unexplained exercise-related deaths occurred in those with sickle cell trait, compared to similar age-, sex-, and race-matched non-sickle cell trait recruits. About half of these deaths were from heat illness, and the other half had no other detectable cause except sickle cell trait.

There is a very rare form of kidney cancer that is sometimes seen in individuals with sickle trait. This is another reason that blood in the urine requires evaluation by a physician.

DIABETES TESTS AND SICKLE CELL TRAIT

If you have sickle cell trait, the hemoglobin A1c test used to diagnose and monitor diabetes may give false low results, which can affect the treatment you receive from your healthcare provider. False low results may mask a high blood sugar, delaying the diagnosis and treatment of diabetes. There are other tests and methods available that will give you accurate results you can trust. Letting your doctor know about your sickle cell trait will help your doctor choose the right test for you. A list of approved tests is available at *www.ngsp.org/interf.asp*.

TRAVEL PRECAUTIONS

The higher you go, the more likely you may be to develop pain or other sickle cell-related problems. People with sickle cell trait may experience trouble when they go to altitudes in excess of 10,000 feet, especially when also experiencing dehydration and heavy exertion—for example, with traveling to cities with high altitudes, such as Mexico City. Car travel in mountain terrains may also cause problems.

Travel in pressurized aircraft usually is fine. Unpressurized aircraft may cause problems at high altitudes.

PREVENTION OF COMPLICATIONS

- The recommendations for exercise in those with sickle cell trait are the same as the general population. When starting a training program, start slow and gradually increase your exercise. Always build up slowly to a desired level of exercise. Don't push the to the limit of your physical endurance.
- Avoid dehydration. Always drink plenty of water and keep a water bottle with you.
- Take rest breaks to allow your body to cool down and recover from exercise.
- If traveling to a high altitude from near sea level, allow a few days to acclimate your body to the pressure and oxygen differences before you undertake physical exertion.

🜉 Avoid exercising in the heat of the day. It is best to walk or run in the morning or evening.

Certain sports are especially risky—for example, mountain climbing to high elevations, sky diving, and skiing at high elevations. Sports and occupations that cause physical exertion in the heat, pressure changes, low oxygen, or dehydration all may cause complications. You should avoid diving with prolonged holding of breath or faulty SCUBA gear.

HAVING CHILDREN

Remember that it is possible for sickle cell disease to occur when one parent has sickle trait, if the other has passed on a gene for another disorder of hemoglobin, such as hemoglobin C, D, E, O, or thalassemia. If both parents are carriers of these genetic combinations, they have a 25% chance of producing a child with sickle cell disease type SC, SD, SE, SO or S beta thalassemia. The risk is 50% if one has sickle cell disease and the other is a carrier.

While prevention is possible, it presents real-life problems of its own. How do you ask the person you just fell in love with to show you his or her genetic map? For that matter, how much thought do most people give to how their genes might damage a child not yet conceived? As you struggle through the problems of an everyday life, such questions may seem far away.

Even people who seek genetic counseling before they plan a family will face emotional and spiritual problems that can become crises. They especially must struggle to decide whether to bring a child into the world, knowing that the child may suffer from sickle cell disease. Any decision one makes can cause guilt. The most important issue is that you and your partner need to know if you carry a gene for sickle hemoglobin or another hemoglobin disorder. A simple blood test can determine if you are at risk. With this information you can make choices based on your risk for have a child with sickle cell disease (See the next two chapters).

To help you increase your knowledge of sickle cell trait, there is a toolkit available for free on the CDC website at *www.cdc.gov/ncbddd/sicklecell/toolkit.html*.

NEW INFORMATION ABOUT SICKLE CELL TRAIT

The journal Annals of Internal Medicine recently published a comprehensive review article by leading sickle cell experts from around the US. They reviewed all of the relevant published evidence about the health outcomes of those with sickle cell trait. This review was led by the Sickle Cell Disease Association of America, the Department of Health and Human Services Secretary's Advisory Committee on Heritable Disorders in Newborns and Children, and the American Society of Hematology to help answer many questions regarding health risks for the estimated 3.5 million Americans and 300 million with sickle cell trait worldwide.

The conclusion of the expert panel was that sickle cell trait is a risk factor for increased risk of pulmonary embolism (blood clots in the legs and lung), kidney disease (Increased urine protein and chronic kidney disease), and exertional rhabdomyolysis (muscle breakdown after exertion), but it does not increase the risk of heart failure, heart attacks, stroke, or decreased growth in children. There was not enough evidence to show any increase in altitude-related spleen infarction or kidney cancer (renal medullary carcinoma).

There are not enough quality published studies that show an increased risk of sudden death with extreme exercise as in the military training or athletics. A large study conducted by the US Army between 2011 and 2014 showed no increase in sudden death in recruits with sickle cell trait. There have been case reports of sudden death in sickle cell trait athletes, but no large controlled studies have been done to determine if increased risk exists.

The authors agree with the American Society of Hematology statement recommending against routine sickle cell trait screening in athletics and support the consistent use of universal precautions to lower exertion-related risk in all persons, regardless of sickle cell trait status. There was moderate-strength evidence that sickle cell trait is a risk factor for exertional rhabdomyolysis, but the risk for that is small, and high-intensity training and genetics may also play a role.

The increased risk for forming blood clots among sickle cell trait carriers compared with non-carriers is at a level similar to that found in other low-risk genetic causes of clotting that do not require screening.

This review helped to answer many questions about sickle cell trait carriers; however, it pointed out the need for more well designed, controlled studies to determine the health risks and methods to lower those risks.

19

Understanding Genetics

GENETICS AND BLOOD DISEASE

Genetics is the science that deals with how plants and animals look and function due to the way genes are expressed. Genes interact with the environment to determine the makeup for every organ, bone, body part, and cell of your body.

Each cell in the human body has a plan, called a *genetic code*, which tells every cell what to make and what to do, much like a house's blueprint. Each unit or part of the code is called a gene. This code is passed from parents to child in the DNA, which is contained in 46 chromosomes. You inherit 23 chromosomes from each parent. You get about one half of most of your genetic code from each of your parents. Your genes determine most of the characteristics that make you unique, things like your gender, eye color, hair color, and skin color. The code also determines your blood type and the types of the hemoglobin inside your red blood cells. A mutation is a change in the DNA code that can cause genetic diseases. This is very much like what would happen if the plan for a house is wrong. If a house plan tells the builder to put a door where a water pipe should go, water would leak everywhere. If the house plan doesn't have enough girders to hold up the house, it could collapse.

HEMOGLOBIN TYPES AND HEMOGLOBINOPATHIES

Hemoglobin is the protein in the red blood cell that carries oxygen from the lungs to the rest of the body and carbon dioxide back to the lungs. It's what makes the blood red. There are normally three types of hemoglobin inside each of the red cells: hemoglobin A (97%), hemoglobin F (1%), and hemoglobin A2 (2%). Your hemoglobin types are genetically determined by the code on chromosomes 16 and 11. The types of hemoglobin you have in your red blood cells can be determined by a simple blood test called hemoglobin electrophoresis. *Hemoglobinopathies* are a group of genetic diseases that occur because of a mutation that causes a small change in the hemoglobin that can affect the way it works. There are more than 900 hemoglobin mutations, but most do not cause any problems.

The substitution of the amino acid valine for glutamic acid in the sixth position of the beta chain coded on chromosome 11 causes the most important mutation: sickle hemoglobin, or Hb S. There are other important mutations such as hemoglobin C, hemoglobin D, hemoglobin E, and hemoglobin O that can interact with sickle hemoglobin to cause the different sickle cell disease types SC, SD, SE, and SO. Because hemoglobin carries oxygen to all parts of the body, the health of the hemoglobin determines the health of the body. Sickle hemoglobin is not healthy because it does not work normally after it gives up oxygen.

Thalassemias are another type of genetic hemoglobin problem. Thalassemia is an inherited hemoglobin problem in which not enough of the subunits that make up the hemoglobin structure are produced. Each hemoglobin molecule is made up of four subunits. In hemoglobin A there are 2 alpha subunits (alpha chains) and two beta subunits (beta chains). Alpha thalassemia occurs if not enough alpha chains are made, and beta thalassemia occurs if not enough beta chains are produced. Thalassemia may be missed in a parent if the hemoglobin electrophoresis is near normal. The best screening for thalassemia is an electronic complete blood count where the mean corpuscular hemoglobin (MCV) is low and the red cell count is elevated.

Most hemoglobin mutations must be inherited from both parents before they cause a disease. It is possible to carry one abnormal hemoglobin gene and one normal hemoglobin gene and not know about it because it does not show itself as disease. This is called a *carrier* state for the disease, also called sickle cell trait.

Sickle Cell Anemia (Hemoglobin SS Disease)
Sickle cell anemia occurs when a child inherits a gene for hemoglobin S from each parent. Either parent may have sickle trait, both may have a sickle cell disease, or one may have sickle cell trait and the other a sickle cell disease. Sickle cell anemia is a serious disease resulting in anemia, increased infection, organ damage, and pain episodes. (See Chapter 2 for more details.)

Hemoglobin SC Disease
Having the sickle cell trait can allow different combinations to form with other abnormal hemoglobins. In hemoglobin SC disease, the Hb S gene is inherited from one parent and the Hb C gene from the other parent. Hemoglobin SC disease is very much like sickle cell disease SS, but milder in some respects with less anemia, fewer problems in childhood, and a better life expectancy. (See Chapter 2 for more details.)

Other Hemoglobins Causing Sickle Cell Disease
There are a number of different hemoglobins that can interact with hemoglobin S to form different types of sickle cell disease These include D, O-Arab, E, and many others. These occur in higher frequency in some parts of the World. For example, hemoglobin E is common in Southeast Asia. Hemoglobin SE disease is rare in most parts of the US but may be seen in populations of immigrants from Southeast Asia, where the disease originated. This is reported to be a milder form of sickle cell disease. (See Chapter 2 for more details.)

Thalassemias and Sickle Beta Thalassemia
Genes causing thalassemia cause decreased or absent production of one or more of the globin chains that make up hemoglobin. They cause a disease in which the red blood cells are too small and do not have enough hemoglobin. Inheriting a beta thalassemia gene with a sickle hemoglobin gene causes a type of sickle cell disease called sickle beta thalassemia. Sickle β^0 thalassemia results when the thalassemia gene causes no beta chain production. This disease is very similar to sickle cell anemia (Hb SS disease) because there is no hemoglobin A in the red cell. Sickle β^+ thalassemia results when the thalassemia gene causes some beta chain production, but not enough. This disease is usually milder than sickle cell anemia because there is some hemoglobin A in the red blood cells.

Alpha thalassemias are caused by genes that affect production of the alpha chain of hemoglobin. Alpha thalassemia genes are common in many populations around the world. They can be inherited with sickle cell diseases and can reduce the severity of many sickle complications.

BLOOD TYPES
Red blood cells have genetically determined proteins, sugars, and type of fats on the outside called *antigens*. These antigens determine the blood type

of the individual. The main blood types are A, B, AB, and O. This blood type remains the same your entire life. There is another antigen, the Rh (Rhesus). If this is present, it will add a label of + or, if absent, a -. Your blood type may be A+, which means type "A with Rh positive, or A-, which means type A Rh negative. There are a large number of other antigens, called minor antigens on your blood cells. These are important when you need to get a blood transfusion.

Individuals will have antibodies against the major blood group antigens if they lack the antigen on their cells—that is, if you have A on your cells, you will have antibody to B, and if you have B, you will make antibody to A. If you have neither, you are type O and will have antibody to A and B. If you are type AB, you will not have antibody to A or B. If you are given a transfusion of red blood cells with an antigen that you have an antibody to, your body will rapidly destroy them and you will have an immediate life-threatening major transfusion reaction. If you lack a minor antigen, you may develop antibodies to red cells with that antigen if you were exposed to red cells with that antigen by past transfusions or pregnancy. If you have antibodies to a minor antigen and are given red cells with that antigen, your body will destroy the transfused cells somewhat later, causing a delayed transfusion reaction.

The blood bank will be very careful to match a unit of donor blood that is compatible with your blood type. If the match is not correct, you could have a transfusion reaction, in which your body attacks the donor red cells. There are a number of minor red blood cell antigens such as Kell, Duffy, Diego, Kidd, and others that are important when transfusing individuals with sickle cell disease. If you are exposed to several blood units over time, you may develop antibodies to many different antigens and have frequent transfusion reactions. To avoid this, the blood bank will try to match the antigens on your red cells to the antigens on the donor red cells to avoid developing the antibodies. This is called phenotypic matching. Another way to prevent this is to minimize your exposure to multiple blood donors. Laura Dean's "Blood Groups and Red Cell Antigens," a good free online book on this subject, is available at *www.ncbi.nlm.nih.gov/books/NBK2261*.

OTHER GENETIC INFLUENCES ON TREATMENT

Another way your genetic code may affect your treatment is how you break down medications in your body. We know there are genetic differences in how the liver works. The liver has systems to activate or break them down many medications. Genetic changes in how the liver does this can cause many medications, especially the opiate class of pain medications widely used for sickle cell pain events, to not work as well or last longer or shorter in the blood. Some people will respond to small amounts of medication, while others require larger doses to get the same pain-fighting effect. There is research underway to see if we can customize the best pain treatments based on your genetic code.

20

Genetic Counseling

By wisdom a house is built, and through understanding it is established.
—*Proverbs 24:3*

THE AIMS OF GENETIC COUNSELING

There is no cure for sickle cell anemia today except through bone marrow transplants. The outlook for individuals with the disease is good and improving constantly, but sickle cell disease is a serious disease with lifelong challenges for the individual and their family. Carriers and those with the disease are at high risk of having a child affected by the disease. A couple who wishes to have children can learn in advance whether their child will have sickle cell disease or be a carrier.

With that knowledge, they can prepare for the serious undertaking of raising a child with this lifelong disease. They can also consider the hard question of whether or not to bring into the world a child likely to suffer with sickle cell disease. Knowing your risk empowers you to make informed decisions.

The Role of a Genetic Counselor

A genetic counselor first:

- learns the medical history of both parents
- takes a detailed family history to determine if genetic diseases are present
- orders blood tests to identify hemoglobinopathy and thalassemia carriers
- may order DNA analyses to confirm the mutation.

Based on this information, the counselor can then determine the chances that the parents will pass on a gene with a mutation to their offspring.

Genetic Counseling

Here Is an Outline of What the Screening Tests May Tell the Counselor and the Parents

Case #	Parent #1	Parent #2	Children*
1	Sickle cell disease Hb SS	Sickle cell disease Hb SS	100% of children → sickle cell disease Hb SS
2	Sickle cell disease Hb SS	Sickle cell trait Hb AS	50% → sickle cell trait Hb AS
			50% → sickle cell disease Hb SS
3	Sickle cell disease Hb SC	Normal Hb AA	50% → trait Hb AS
			50% → trait Hb AC
4	Normal Hb AA	Normal Hb AA	100% → normal Hb AA
5	Sickle cell trait Hb AS	Sickle cell trait Hb AS	25% → normal Hb AA
			50% → trait Hb AS
			25% → disease Hb SS
6	Sickle cell trait Hb AS	Normal Hb AA	50% → trait Hb AS
			50% → normal Hb AA
7	Sickle cell trait Hb AS	Hemoglobin-C trait Hb AC	25% → trait Hb AS
			25% → trait Hb AC
			25% → normal Hb AA
			25% → disease Hb SC
8	Sickle cell trait Hb AS	Beta thalassemia trait	25% → trait AS
			25% → beta thal trait
			25% → normal Hb AA
			25% → disease S beta thal

*Percent (%) represents the chances of hemoglobin pattern each child may have with each pregnancy

SCT and Genetics

Ideally, the genetic counselor can explain the risk of having an affected child before conception so the parents know the risks. They may also help the parents understand testing that is available during the pregnancy to determine before birth if the child is affected. If there is a chance that the couple will pass on sickle cell disease to a baby, the counselor will talk to the parents about the resources they will need to raise a child with sickle cell disease. The counselor will also describe the effect the disease is likely to have on the parents' lives as well as the child's.

Besides informing prospective parents whether they are likely to pass on the gene with a mutation, the genetic counselor helps after the baby is born by ordering tests that allow precise diagnosis. Genetic counselors often participate in confirming the diagnosis in the infant, determining the risks in future pregnancies, and identifying other family members who may be at risk for having a child with sickle cell disease.

Finding and Working With a Genetic Counselor

Many major universities have genetics programs with certified genetic counselors. University hospitals are usually good sources of information because they are affiliated with medical schools that have genetic counselors and a full range of genetic diagnostic services.

Your primary care doctor or specialist can direct you to a nearby university hospital that provides genetic services.

Many local community-based sickle cell organizations provide reproductive education and genetic counseling focused on sickle cell disease. They may provide or know of sources for genetic counseling in your community.

All states now screen all newborns for sickle cell disease shortly after birth. The primary reason for screening is to detect sickle cell disease early so infants can receive healthcare and start penicillin to prevent early deaths from infection. These screening programs also detect large numbers of infants who are carriers for Hb S and other abnormal hemoglobins. Most have excellent follow-up programs for testing, education, and counseling of the parents of these infants. You can find a genetic counselor by contacting your local health department as well as state genetic services coordinators who are part of these programs.

You may also contact your state or county's medical society, or any of the organizations listed in the Resources section, for referrals to university hospitals. The National Society of Genetic Counselors website can help you find a counselor at *www.nsgc.org*.

PARENTS' OPTIONS

A counselor can help determine the odds, but only the parents can decide whether to bring into the world a child who may have sickle cell disease. Some couples would rather not risk having children who are likely to be born with sickle cell disease. Such a couple has three options:

- avoid pregnancy completely;
- have the baby only when they know, through prenatal tests, that the fetus is perfectly healthy;
- request preimplantation genetic diagnosis (PGD) to only proceed with the pregnancy if the fetus does not have sickle cell disease. Many infertility clinics now offer these services.

Avoiding Pregnancy

Avoiding pregnancy is the simplest and least expensive option. It is also safest for the mother, although a couple may naturally feel emotional pain knowing they can never have their own biological child. Even if an individual wants to have a child who may have sickle cell disease, it is very wise to delay pregnancy until one is in a stable relationship with good support systems. Raising a child with sickle cell disease can be very challenging and requires lots of help.

Couples have several ways of avoiding pregnancy:

- Abstinence from all sex that could result in pregnancy.
- Contraceptives, such as condoms or foams, are readily available at the local drug store. Remember that it takes only one incident of unprotected sex to impregnate a woman. Because the choices are difficult once the woman is pregnant, couples should talk frankly with one another about the importance of contraception. Condoms also provide good protection against sexually transmitted diseases.
- Contraceptive pills, implants, IUDs and other forms of contraception are widely available and very effective in preventing pregnancy. Most do not protect against sexually transmitted diseases. Consult your primary physician, gynecologist, or family planning clinic to determine which method is best for you.

- Another method of avoiding pregnancy is sterilization. The male can undergo a vasectomy, which is the tying of the tubes that allow sperm to move from the testes to the penis. The female may have her fallopian tubes (the organs in which the eggs are fertilized) tied. Neither operation affects sexual performance. Both are usually very difficult to reverse.

Adoption is always an option for couples who are reluctant to have a child affected by sickle cell disease. There are many children available who need loving homes.

Aborting All But Healthy Fetuses
The second option is to have the baby *only* if tests determine that the fetus is healthy. This option may create new obstacles for the couple.

One obstacle is religion. Abortion is prohibited by the Islamic religion and the Roman Catholic Church. Many religions and churches also discourage or forbid abortion. It is not permitted in Orthodox Judaism, with several exceptions. Religion aside, many women and many men feel that it is morally wrong to abort the fetus at any stage of the pregnancy.

Legal restrictions on abortion may also pose difficulties. While abortion has been legal in all states since 1973, many states have recently placed restrictions on them. If this is an option for you, ask your doctor or legal advisor about the abortion laws in your state.

Detection of Sickle Cell Disease Through Prenatal Testing
The prenatal tests that diagnose birth defects, including sickle cell disease, are amniocentesis and chorionic villus sampling. Both are widely available and each has risks and benefits. These can be used to determine if a child is affected in case the parents are considering terminating the pregnancy. More commonly, they are used to determine if a child is affected so that the parents can be reassured or start preparing to raise the child with disease.

Amniocentesis is performed under local anesthesia by inserting a large needle through the abdomen in order to withdraw a small amount of the amniotic fluid. The sample fluid contains cells from the fetus that can be grown and whose DNA can then be analyzed. This procedure can be done only in the sixteenth through the eighteenth weeks of pregnancy, and the results take two to three weeks.

This means that the woman will be well into her pregnancy before she can be tested and get results. Because the test must be done fairly late, there may not be time to consider an abortion if that is an option. The woman also faces some risks from the sampling procedure itself.

Another procedure for prenatal diagnosis is *chorionic villus sampling* (CVS). This can be performed somewhat earlier, at twelve to fourteen weeks, and the results can be seen within 48 hours. However, the faster procedure carries 1%–2% or greater risk of miscarriage, and there are concerns that it can cause birth defects. Furthermore, the test is less accurate. This means there is a higher possibility that some women, on the basis of this test, might abort babies who would have been perfectly healthy, or have an unanticipated baby with disease.

Preimplantation Genetic Diagnosis
The third option for a couple that has decided not to risk having a child born with sickle cell disease is *preimplantation genetic diagnosis* (PGD). PGD is an option for some parents because it doesn't require them to decide to abort the fetus if it will be born with sickle cell disease. This procedure involves taking eggs from the woman's ovary *before* she is pregnant and fertilizing them in a laboratory dish (in vitro fertilization). When the fertilized eggs begin to divide, one of the cells is taken out for DNA analysis and tested for sickle cell anemia and any other genetic disease. If the embryo is genetically normal, it is implanted into the mother, who completes the pregnancy. If it has the disease, the embryo is discarded. Infertility clinics would be the best resource for PGD.

PROSPECTS FOR THE FUTURE

Today the genetic counselor's primary role is to provide information about genetic diseases and available resources, predict the likelihood of a healthy baby, and inform the parents of the options available to them.

In the future, the counselor may be part of a team that might be able to do much more.

Researchers are working on gene therapy solutions that have been successful in correcting the sickle cell mutation in stem cells. These methods could theoretically be used to correct the mutation in a single fertilized cell, correcting the disease before implantation. However, there are considerable practical, legal, and ethical problems to overcome before this method can be considered for use on humans. (See Chapter 15.)

SUMMING IT UP

Genetic testing and counseling provides all individuals who are at risk for sickle cell disease to understand their risks. There are a number of options available to determine if a child will be born with sickle cell disease, providing numerous opportunities to control that risk. With these opportunities come very hard choices.

But knowledge is of little value if we don't act on it. Let's listen to one couple hashing out their problem with friends. The couple is Derrick and Laquana, and they've just been told by their genetic counselor that they each carry the sickle cell trait and that they have one chance in four of having a child with sickle cell disease. The other couple, Keeshawn and Shaniqua, haven't yet been tested, but they plan to be. Laquana opens the discussion.

DERRICK AND LAQUANA'S STORY

Laquana: Derrick and I went to the doctor last week to get tested for sickle trait and other hemoglobin problems.

Derrick: Yeah, turns out we both have sickle trait.

Keeshawn: Have you decided what you'll do?

Laquana: We've thought it over a lot. Derrick wants a child, and says he's ready to be a really involved father. And you know, for me… well, we ladies do have that biological clock that keeps ticking. And I'm at the point in my career now where I can take some time off without risking my job. So we've decided to have a child.

Shaniqua: Congratulations! I'm scared about the possibility of having a child with sickle cell disease. It's hard enough to raise a normal child.

Derrick: We know it's no piece of cake. But from what the doctor told us and stuff we've been reading off the Internet, the outlook for kids with sickle cell disease is a lot better than it used to be. There are new treatments, better ways to prevent crises, even occasional cures with bone marrow transplant, and a lot more support out there for families.

Shaniqua: You know me—I have to be blunt: I just don't think its right to bring another child into the world with a chronic illness if we can help it.

Keeshawn: Yeah, that's my feeling too. Shaniqua and I have decided that, when she gets pregnant, we'll have prenatal testing. If the fetus tests positive for sickle cell disease, she'll have an abortion. It's not fair to bring a child into the world who's going to suffer so much, and who might have a shorter life after all that suffering.

Shaniqua: Yes. If we decide that we can't have a biological child, there are so many kids in the world who need a loving home. We can adopt one.

Laquana: Well, there you are. We feel that abortion is something we can't handle. Derrick and I will also have prenatal testing, but if the fetus tests positive for sickle cell disease, we're going to use the rest of the pregnancy to learn as much as we can about the disease and that way give our child the longest, healthiest, happiest life possible.

Derrick: That's right. We know it won't be easy, but we've thought about it a lot. If the baby is born with sickle cell, she is going to get the best loving and caring any baby can get.

Derrick and Laquana Have Their Child

Derrick and Laquana went through with the plan they talked about. Throughout Laquana's pregnancy, she was carefully monitored by the pediatrician. Now the baby, Booker, is three months old and has sickle cell disease type SS. At their pediatrician's recommendation, they regularly see a pediatric hematologist at University Medical Center. They are very happy with their new pediatrician. Derrick and Laquana bring her their questions, and she takes time to explain things.

SUPPORT AND NETWORKING

As long as children with sickle cell disease do come into the world, they deserve to get the best, most loving care. By drawing on the education, support, and networking other people can provide, parents can anticipate problems and deal with them before they get too big.

One of a parent's first obligations is to know what to expect at each stage of a child's illness and to recognize problems at their earliest stages, when they can be dealt with most effectively. Managing a disease means knowing the best ways to avoid a serious outbreak of symptoms or still more serious complications. Knowing what to expect, not being caught off guard, means the parent can react earlier, in a calmer frame of mind, and prevent some emergencies.

Resources

FOR INDIVIDUALS WITH SICKLE CELL AND THEIR FAMILIES

CHECK (Coordination of Health Care for Complex Kids)
A program provided by the University of Illinois at Chicago with sickle cell education modules for children and parents.
https://www.mycheck.uic.edu/sickle-cell

Sickle Cell Community Consortium
Composed of community-based sickle cell organizations, patient and caregiver advocates, community partners, and medical and research advisors. The group is active in defining problems and needs of the population and planning and implementing solutions.
http://sicklecellconsortium.org/

"Get Connected" Registry
A clearinghouse of information for sickle cell patients and their families on such topics as advocacy, treatments, therapies, and research. Click on the "Register" button to begin.
www4.gvtsecure.com/reg_scdaa

Sickle Cell Warriors
An online community for sickle cell patients and families.
www.sicklecellwarriors.com

FOR HEALTHCARE PROVIDERS

ASH Pocket Guide App
The American Society of Hematology's series of brief, evidence-based pocket guides is now available in a smartphone app, available for both Android

(in the Google Play store) and iOS devices (in the App Store).

NHLBI Guidelines, 2014
Guidelines and Evidence Tables from the National Heart, Lung, and Blood Institute's Expert Panel Report on Evidence-Based Management of Sickle Cell Disease are available to download from NHLBI's website.
https://www.nhlbi.nih.gov/health-topics/evidence-based-management-sickle-cell-disease

American Pain Society Clinical Practice Guidelines
Evidence-based guidelines for complex pain management cases.
americanpainsociety.org/education/guidelines/overview

FOR FAMILIES, PROVIDERS, AND THE COMMUNITY

Centers for Disease Control and Prevention
Sickle cell information, statistics, tips for healthy living, and other free material from the CDC.
www.cdc.gov/ncbddd/sicklecell/index.html

Sickle Cell Information Center
The leading web-based resource for sickle cell information, founded by *Hope and Destiny* authors James Eckman, MD, and Allan Platt, PA-C, MMSc.
www.scinfo.org

KEY COMMUNITY ORGANIZATIONS AND INFORMATION ON THE WEB

The Internet is an invaluable resource for researching sickle cell support groups. Key organizations, such as the Sickle Cell Disease Association of America (SCDAA), the Foundation for Sickle Cell Disease Research, the American Sickle Cell Anemia Association (ASCAA), and the Sickle Cell Information Center, have links nationwide. The Sickle Cell Society is based in London, England, to help patients and families in Europe. The Nigerian Society for Sickle Cell is an umbrella group that seeks to unite the efforts in Nigeria. Sickle Cell Warriors grew from a social media community to an actual organization. Other popular social media groups are Sickle Cell United and Sickle Cell 101. All of these groups are working to raise awareness of the needs of the sickle cell patient while reaching out to patients and families.

> ## Medical Information on the Internet
>
> There are hundreds of websites offering medical information on the Internet. Many sites offer wonderful information, while other sites do not. You need to judge the credibility of the information on the Internet by using a few simple rules:
>
> - Who is the author of the information? You can look at the last three letters of the website and see *.gov* for US government sites like *NIH.gov* and *CDC.gov*. Those ending in *.edu* are sponsored by educational institutes like universities. Those ending in *.org* are usually non-profit organizations.
>
> - Is there an editorial board that oversees the information? This should include physicians and other healthcare providers.
>
> - Is the site selling you a medication or treatment? Are there excessive commercials within the site? Be wary of bias in the information.
>
> - Is the information current? Check the dates of the information.
>
> - Is your privacy being protected? Be wary of sites that want too much personal information before they give you information.
>
> - See if the website is a member of Health on the Net (HON): *www.hon.ch/HONcode*.

Sickle Cell Warriors

"A site for those Learning Loving, Living, Achieving, Caring, Righting, and Surviving Sickle Cell Disease." Online community for information and support, guided by Tosin Ola, a nurse and a mother. The virtual community recently started annual face-to-face meetings on a cruise ship. *sicklecellwarriors.com*

Sickle Cell Information Center

This is a comprehensive sickle cell site based at Emory University in Atlanta, Georgia. In 1984, Grady Memorial Hospital opened the world's first 24-hour comprehensive acute care sickle cell center. The goals of the center were to provide 24-hour acute care in a designated area with a dedicated staff, provide healthcare consultations, research new treatments, and provide education and support services to residents of the state of Georgia with sickle cell syndromes. Upgraded in 2016, the mission of the website continues to be providing sickle cell patients and professionals with education, news, research updates, and worldwide sickle cell resources. E-mail consultations are now provided to patients and clinicians in countries around the world. All e-mail questions are reviewed by a physician assistant and answered or sent to the appropriate medical staff member for a reply.

The website contains a section for healthcare providers, including an overview of the disease, two online clinical-management books, research updates, conference information, Web links, and news. There is also a section for patients and family members contain articles in lay terms, a frequently-asked-questions page, downloadable educational coloring books, means of submitting e-mail questions, and locations of sickle cell clinics nationwide. Also found on the website is an extensive list of links to other sickle cell websites; a resource page with recommended books, videos, monographs, and CD-ROMs; information on worldwide sickle cell educational conferences; and an informational guide for teachers and employers to help sickle cell patients with basic pain-prevention measures. On the News page, patients, family members, and healthcare providers can subscribe to a free monthly e-mail newsletter.
www.scinfo.org

Globin Gene Server
This site provides data and tools for studying the function of DNA sequences, with an emphasis on those involved in the production of hemoglobin. There is an online copy of *A Syllabus of Human Hemoglobin Variants* (1996) and most of *A Syllabus of Thalassemia Mutations* (1997).
globin.cse.psu.edu

Centers for Disease Control (CDC) Sickle Cell Information Web Page
This site has sickle cell information on incidence and prevention of complications, up-to-date information on sickle trait, and a guide to sickle cell organizations and facilities.

Centers for Disease Control
1600 Clifton Road
Atlanta, GA 30329
800-232-4636; *www.cdc.gov/ncbddd/sicklecell/index.html*

Medscape
This site features an electronic medical textbook chapter on sickle cell pain crisis written for healthcare professionals; it has excellent information.
https://emedicine.medscape.com/article/205926-overview

Genetics Home Reference
This site presents information from the NIH on sickle cell disease.
ghr.nlm.nih.gov/condition/sickle-cell-disease

Sickle Cell Kids
This is a kid-friendly site full of sickle cell information in a fun, animated presentation. There are games, stories, letters from celebrities, and more. The staff of the Sickle Cell Center in Atlanta provides the scientific content.
www.SickleCellKids.org

Harvard School of Medicine Information Center for Sickle Cell and Thalassemic Disorders
This excellent site has information for clinicians and patients. There are very good articles about current issues in sickle cell treatment and links to other sickle cell sites.
sickle.bwh.harvard.edu/index.html

March of Dimes
Information on sickle cell disease as it relates to pregnancy and newborns can be found on the March of Dimes website.
www.marchofdimes.org/complications/sickle-cell-disease-and-pregnancy.aspx
www.marchofdimes.org/complications/sickle-cell-disease-and-your-baby.aspx

National Library of Medicine
You can search MEDLINE for free and access the latest publications in the medical press. There are free journal abstracts and many free full-text articles.
www.ncbi.nlm.nih.gov/pubmed

MedlinePlus—Sickle Cell Anemia
This site offers an overview of sickle cell disease in terms that the layperson can understand, with many links to sites with additional information.
www.nlm.nih.gov/medlineplus/sicklecellanemia.html

NATIONAL AND INTERNATIONAL ORGANIZATIONS

From 1972 to 2008, the National Institutes of Health (NIH) funded Comprehensive Sickle Cell Centers (CSCCs) as model programs that enhanced sickle cell services with clinical research and community services such as screening, counseling, and education.

Ten CSCCs were funded at a time, and the list of centers would change every five years because of the federal government's funding cycles. The NIH stopped funding the CSCCs in April 2008. About thirty medical centers still follow the comprehensive sickle cell centers model. Clinical research continues, and is organized in several overlapping networks of these sickle cell centers. However, the support for the community services like screening, counseling, and education is uncertain. A list of clinics is maintained at the CDC Sickle cell website: *www.cdc.gov/ncbddd/sicklecell/map/map-nationalresourcedirectory.html*

The Sickle Cell Disease Association of America

The goal of the Sickle Cell Disease Association of America (SCDAA) is "to find a cure and improve the quality of life for those who are afflicted and their families." The SCDAA publishes and distributes to parents and teachers educational materials for living and coping with sickle cell disease.

Through its member organizations, SCDAA provides such services as screening and referrals, counseling, home nursing care, research updates, psychosocial services, transportation, summer camp, local and regional workshops, international symposia, as well as a sickle cell chat room. The SCDAA also provides guidelines for starting local sickle cell groups.

Sickle Cell Disease Association of America
3700 Koppers Street
Suite 570
Baltimore, MD 21227
800-421-8453
410-528-1555
410-528-1495 fax
www.sicklecelldisease.org
E-mail: admin@sicklecelldisease.org

Foundation for Sickle Cell Disease Research (FSCDR)
Hosts an annual scientific exposition focused on sickle cell disease. Community members and patients are welcome to mingle with research scientists, government officials, pharmaceutical companies, physicians and other healthcare providers.

3858 Sheridan Street
Suite S
Hollywood, FL 33021
954-397-3251
info@fscdr.org
https://fscdr.org

The American Society of Hematology
This is the national organization supporting hematologists (blood experts). They support sickle cell research, publications, and professional education. They have an annual meeting at which many sickle cell research results are presented.

American Society of Hematology
2021 L Street NW
Suite 900
Washington, DC 20036
202-776-0544
202-776-0545 fax
www.hematology.org

The Sickle Cell Society of London, England
This is an international sickle cell organization based in England that supports patient and professional education.

Sickle Cell Society
54 Station Road
London
NW10 4UA
UK
020-8961-7795
020-8961-8346 (fax)
www.sicklecellsociety.org

The Alliance of Genetic Support Groups
This nonprofit health-advocacy organization is committed to transforming health through genetics.

The Alliance of Genetic Support Groups
4301 Connecticut Avenue NW
Suite 404
Washington, DC 20008
202-966-5557
202-966-8553 (fax)
www.geneticalliance.org
info@geneticalliance.org

International Association of Sickle Cell Nurses and Physician Assistants (IASCNAPA)
IASCNAPA is an association of nurses, physician assistants, and other healthcare workers caring for sickle cell patients worldwide.
www.iascnapa.org

National Heart, Lung, and Blood Institute (NHLBI)
The NHLBI is a part of the federal government's National Institutes of Health, focused on research, training, and education programs to promote the prevention and treatment of heart, lung, and blood diseases. New 2014 NIH evidence-based sickle cell guidelines aimed for primary care healthcare providers is published at *www.nhlbi.nih.gov/health-pro/guidelines/sickle-cell-disease-guidelines*

Online educational material for community members is available at *www.nhlbi.nih.gov/health/health-topics/topics/sca/*

NHLBI Health Information Center
P.O. Box 30105
Bethesda, MD 20824-0105
301-592-8573
www.nhlbi.nih.gov
nhlbiinfo@nhlbi.nih.gov

St. Jude Children's Research Hospital—Sickle Cell Program
St. Jude's provides comprehensive treatment, conducts research, and provides clinical trials in its sickle cell program. A range of educational materials

for parents, patients, and health educators are available for download at *www.stjude.org/treatment/disease/sickle-cell-disease/educational-resources.html*

A set of videos to help adolescents with sickle cell transition to adulthood are available at *www.stjude.org/treatment/disease/sickle-cell-disease/step-program.html*

St. Jude Children's Research Hospital
262 Danny Thomas Place
Memphis, TN 38105
866-278-5833

www.stjude.org/treatment/disease/sickle-cell-disease.html

The American Pain Society
This organization published "The Guideline for the Management of Acute and Chronic Pain in Sickle-Cell Disease" in 1999 and has many pain-management resources. The review was a landmark evidence-based sickle cell pain guide peer reviewed by many experts in sickle cell disease. Although not incorporating new 21st century research on mechanisms of sickle cell pain, the Guideline is still the only handbook focusing on pain assessment and treatment.

The American Pain Society
8735 W. Higgins Road
Suite 300
Chicago, IL 60631
847-375 4715
www.ampainsoc.org
info@americanpainsociety.org

VIDEOS

YouTube
This online community offers many free educational videos about sickle cell disease and trait. Just type in "sickle cell" in the search box. Any individual can post a video on this site, so it is a powerful way to share your message. Like anything on the Internet, you must be wary of the sources you watch.

BOOKS AND BOOKLETS

Hope and Destiny Jr.—The Adolescent's Guide to Sickle Cell Disease by Lewis Hsu, MD, Silvia Brandalise, MD, and Carmen Rodrigues, RN

The best resource available today for young patients and families impacted by sickle cell disease. It is the only comprehensive, educational book on the market written especially for children that tackles all aspects of the disease.
https://hiltonpub.com/bookstore/

Hope and Destiny Jr. Workbook by Lewis Hsu, MD

A streamlined version of *Hope and Destiny Jr.*, plus some added educational puzzles, written for children in their "tweens."
https://hiltonpub.com/bookstore/

Sickle What? by Lisa Rose, Hilton Publishing. 2016.

This is a booklet for parents of a baby who has just been diagnosed with sickle cell. In clear simple language plus pictures, it provides the basics of home care for sickle cell, written by a mother who is also an educator.
https://hiltonpub.com/bookstore/

Living with Sickle Cell: The Inside Story by Judy Gray Johnson

Describes the way sickle cell disease affects different systems in the body. Based on first-hand experience by the author, herself a sickle cell patient.
www.knowledgepowerinc.com/Sickle_Cell.html

Understanding Sickle Cell Disease by Miriam Bloom, PhD

This is an excellent book written for lay audiences by the former senior editor for the Journal of the National Cancer Institute. The book is well organized and contains current information explaining the origins, complications, treatments, and the future of research for sickle cell disease.
www.sciwrite.com/b_sickle_cell.html.

Sickle Cell Disease, Third Edition, by Graham Serjeant, M.D.

This is one of the most comprehensive medical textbooks in the world. Dr. Serjeant spent much of his medical career caring for sickle cell patients in Jamaica and has traveled around the world as a sickle cell consultant. This text is written for medical personnel, but it is a good reference book to have on the shelf. Oxford Press 2001. ISBN 0-19-263036-9.

Sickle Cell Anemia: From Basic Science to Clinical Practice, edited by Fernando Costa and Nicola Conran.
The most recent reference book for medical professionals. Each chapter is written by two or more expert authors. They present up-to-date summaries from laboratory research ("Basic Science") to patient care ("Clinical Practice"). Elsevier 2016. ISBN 978-3-319-06712-4.

Puzzles by Dava Walker
Puzzles is a story about Cassie, a school-age child with sickle cell disease. This book for children is available from Carolina Wren Press, ISBN 0-914996-29-0. There is a discount for schools, hospitals, clinics, libraries, and other nonprofit agencies; contact publisher for details.
carolinawrenpress.org.

Renaissance of Sickle Cell Disease Research in the Genome Era edited by Betty S. Pace
This is a wonderful text book for clinical and basic researchers in hematology and genetics, graduate students and postdoctoral fellows, and may also be of interest to nursing students, community sickle cell programs, medical school libraries, public library. It has several great authors who are the leaders in sickle cell research and treatment. This book is great for anyone wanting to know the current state of sickle cell disease research. University of Texas at Dallas, ISBN 978-1-86094-645-5.
www.worldscientific.com/worldscibooks/10.1142/p443

Sickle by Dominique Friend
Sickle is a book written by Dominique Friend about her personal experiences living with sickle cell disease. Its purpose is to encourage, uplift, and bring forth awareness of a disease that affects almost 1 in 500 African Americans. Dominique has captured in writing the very essence of what it is like to find purpose in spite of pain, transfusions, medicines, and emergency room visits. Her story will inspire others to speak out and gain confidence "that the battle against this disease does go on." This book is truly a must-have for all those affected by sickle cell disease. ISBN 978-0-61526-546-9.

Now You See Me, Now You Don't by Jan Reed-Givhan
This is a moving and inspiring novel about a young black girl's battle with racial discrimination as well as sickle cell anemia. Based upon a true story, this book poignantly reveals what challenges a teenage girl can face growing

up with a terrible disease in a sometimes emotionally unhealthy environment. Her story pulls no punches, and yet offers greater understanding and hope. ISBN 978-1-41963-247-1.

Sickle Cell Pain, second edition, by Samir K. Ballas.
Dr. Ballas draws upon decades of experience taking care of adults with sickle cell in Philadelphia and as a respected researcher to provide a panoramic, in-depth exploration of the multiple dimensions of sickle cell disease: scientific, human, and social. This is a unique book as the only comprehensive, definitive work devoted to sickle cell pain, as opposed to general aspects of the disease. ISBN 978-0-931092-06-0.
ebooks.iasp-pain.org/sickle_cell_pain

Sickle Cell Disease—A Booklet for Patients, Parents, and the Community by Dr. Adlette Inati Khoriaty
The objective of this booklet is to provide families of patients affected with sickle cell disease with accurate and concise information about this disease to help them give their children the best treatment possible. This booklet is also meant to enable parents to actively share with their physicians in the care of their children and often suspect the diagnosis of devastating complications and seek help at an early age. It will also help parents handle the disease and teach them ways of dealing with their children in a positive, supportive, and disciplined manner. In addition, this booklet will provide older patients with concise and simplistic information about coping with the disease and its complications.
issuu.com/internationalthalassaemiafederation/docs/scd_english.

Uncertain Suffering: Racial Health Care Disparities and Sickle Cell Disease (George Gund Foundation Imprint in African-American Studies), by Carolyn Moxley Rouse
This book provides a richly nuanced examination of what race disparities mean for health care in the United States. Through the lens of sickle cell anemia, Rouse argues that resources should be redirected to community-based health programs that reduce daily forms of physical and mental suffering. Available through University of California Press at *www.ucpress.edu*. ISBN 978-0-52025-912-6.

Menace in My Blood: My Affliction with Sickle Cell Anemia, by Ola Tamedu
Tamedu relates growing up in a fairly well-to-do family in West Africa and highlights the difficulties of life with sickle cell disease. 187 pages; ISBN 1-4120-5017-0.
https://www.trafford.com/bookstore/bookdetail.aspx?bookid=SKU-000150130

A Sick Life: TLC 'n Me: Stories from On and Off the Stage, by Tionne Watkins (T-Boz)
As the lead singer of Grammy-winning supergroup TLC, Tionne "T-Boz" Watkins has seen phenomenal fame, success, and critical acclaim. But backstage, she has lived a dual life. In addition to the balancing act of juggling an all-consuming music career and her family, Tionne has struggled her whole life with sickle-cell disease—a debilitating and incurable condition that can render her unable to perform, walk, or even breathe. Rodale Press, 2017. 256 pages; ISBN 978-1-63565-212-3.

A Doctor in a Patient's Body: Dreaming Big with Sickle Cell Disease and Chronic Pain, by Dr. Simone Eastman Uwan
This book shows by example that people with chronic pain and a lifelong disease can still make a powerful impact if they follow their calling. To quote Dr. Uwan, "I'm a sickle cell thriver, not just a survivor!"
http://www.facebook.com/simone.eastmanuwan

Dying in the City of Blues: Sickle Cell Anemia and the Politics of Race and Health, by Keith Wailoo
This is a 360-page description of the history, social, cultural, and political aspects of sickle cell disease in Memphis, TN. University of North Carolina Press, 2001.
uncpress.unc.edu/books/T-4855.html

SCHOOL GUIDES AND PARENT GUIDES

Timberly's Story
https://hiltonpub.com/bookstore/

Educator's Guide to Sickle Cell and School, Parents Guide to Sickle Cell, Children's Mercy Hospital, Kansas City, MO.
www.childrensmercy.org/sickle-cell-disease

Sickle Cell and Thalassaemia—Health and Safety at School, A Guide to School Policy. Simon Dyson.
www.sicklecellanaemia.org

ADOLESCENT TRANSITION GUIDES

Got Transition
Provides information and resources for transition planning for healthcare providers, youth and their families, and researchers and policy makers. They define the six core elements of transition and provide extensive information and tools to assist in transition.
www.gottransition.org

Florida Health and Transition Services (FloridaHATS)
Great source for information on transition for health care practitioners, youth and their families, and others. Excellent tool box provides documents and links to resources that support transition from pediatric to adult-centered care.
www.floridahats.org

Sickle Cell Transition E-Learning Program (STEP) for Teens with Sickle Cell Disease, St. Jude Children's Research Hospital
Booklet and online educational modules
www.stjude.org/treatment/disease/sickle-cell-disease/step-program.html

Sickle Cell Adolescent Transition (SCAT), Children's National Medical Center
Online educational modules
https://childrensnational.org/departments/_resources-for-families/sickle-cell-transition-education-project

Florida Transition Project
For children with disabilities, families, and service-providing community agencies
www.floridatransitionproject.ucf.edu

MEETINGS

There are several national and regional meetings listed on the News page at the Sickle Cell Information website at *www.scinfo.org*. You also can subscribe to the free monthly e-mail newsletters. Some are for patients and families, others are for medical providers, and some offer content for both audiences.

SCDAA

Sickle Cell Disease Association of American hosts an annual convention near its headquarters in Baltimore, Maryland. The convention's goal is to bring together the community-based organizations for sickle cell in many states, healthcare providers, government officials, and the pharmaceutical industry. Workshops, project meetings, and inspirational stories are shared. Practical training occurs for community health workers, nurses, patient advocates, and grassroots advocates. The agenda also include lectures by established leaders and rising stars in the sickle cell community. In addition, SCDAA hosts an annual "Day on Capitol Hill" to build awareness of sickle cell disease among US senators, US congressional representatives, and their legislative staff.

FSCDR

"The Foundation for Sickle Cell Disease Research is committed to supporting innovative research in sickle cell disease to help maximize quality of life and improve survival for the generations of people affected with this disease. An annual conference near its headquarters in Hollywood, Florida, seeks to provide a platform for researchers, healthcare providers, individuals and their families living with sickle cell disease and supporters to work collaboratively in identifying barriers that are limiting creation, adoption and adherence to evidence-based screening recommendations, new therapeutics and best practices that help in the management of sickle cell disease."
fscdr.org/Home/About-Us

Sickle Cell in Focus (SCIF)

An annual meeting that alternates between London, England, and Bethesda, Maryland, to provide updates for healthcare providers, researchers, patients and families.

Local groups

Most regions with a sizable number of people with sickle disease have community-based organizations or patient advocacy and support group hosted by a medical schools. In many states, these are member organizations of the SCDAA. Look for these groups to host an annual information session, Research Day, or updates about advances in sickle cell care. Other events aim to raise awareness or financial support.

HEALTH PASSPORT

Name: _____

Date of birth: _____

Sickle cell type: _____

Medical record number: _____

Allergies: _____

Medications: _____

Physician: _____

Physician's phone number: _____

Complications: _____

_____

Transfusions: _____

_____

Transfusion problems or alloantibodies?   yes / no

Blood bank that has my records: _____

Surgeries: _____

_____

Pain medications: _____

_____

ER pain medications: _____

_____

Immunizations: _____

_____

_____

CLINICS

The national and international list of clinics with sickle cell services is growing daily. Please check the latest national resource directory on the CDC's sickle cell website.

www.cdc.gov/ncbddd/sicklecell/map/map-nationalresourcedirectory.html

If you cannot find a clinic near you, ask other patients and supporters about where they obtain good medical care. If you have no patients or sickle cell associations to ask, start with the nearest hematologist, followed by your pediatrician. It is worthwhile to establish annual contact with a large sickle cell center to keep informed about the latest advances and have an established relationship if you have a complicated problem.

SCHOLARSHIPS

A state-by-state listing of member chapters where you can obtain local chapter scholarship information is located at *www.sicklecelldisease.org*.

SMARTPHONE APPS

Pinpoint App—By providing information about SCD including causes, treatments, and care options, Pinpoint can improve self-care and communication skills for teens through a technology with which they're accustomed and use daily. *Currently under development for iPhones and Android devices.*

VOICE Crisis Alert allows you to track your symptoms and pain and share them with your family members and healthcare providers. *Available in the App Store and Google Play Store.*

Sickle Cell Iron Invaders is a game that takes you on an exciting adventure through the body, with information about sickle cell along the way. *Available in the App Store.*

POMS: Prevention of Morbidity in Sickle Cell Anemia allows you to keep track of your sickle cell pain. *Available in the App Store.*

Sickle-O-Scope is a diary to record your symptoms, with visualizations of your condition. You can share the data you collect with your healthcare provider. *Available in the App Store and Google Play Store.*

Sickle Buddy is an app for children to learn and live with sickle cell disease. *Available in the App Store.*

SCD Toolbox is an app for adults and includes medical guides. *Available in the App Store.*

SCD Share is an app to increase awareness and knowledge of sickle disease. *Available in the App Store.*

Little George is an informational game about sickle cell anemia for children and young people. Pay a visit to Waggle Avenue where Little George learns how to manage his pain during a sickle cell crisis, with help from his mum and his friend Dragon along the way. This application has been inspired by patients at Alder Hey Children's NHS Foundation Trust. *Available in the App Store.*

THE HISTORY OF SICKLE CELL DISEASE

Background

Hemoglobinopathies are a group of genetic diseases that occur because of a mutation in the DNA blueprint that directs the making of hemoglobin. Hemoglobin is important because it is the main carrier of oxygen in the body. Only 1 percent of the wide variety of hemoglobinopathies can cause serious diseases such as sickle cell disease and the thalassemias. Thus, you and I can carry a hemoglobin gene abnormality and not know about it because it does not show itself as disease.

Sometimes we take knowledge for granted without honoring the human effort that went into gaining it. Let's correct that by going back in time to see how we learned that hemoglobinopathies are inherited from our parents.

The story begins in the 19th century, when a simple but very damaging blood disorder called *hemophilia* plagued royal families, though only the males were afflicted by it. Hemophilia leads to massive bleeding when an injury occurs inside or outside the body. Without treatment, the hemophiliac can die of bleeding from even minor wounds.

Treatment for hemophilia means transfusion, but blood transfusion wasn't available at this time. And without the benefits of transfusion, most hemophiliacs, even royal ones, easily bled to death.

In 1865, an Austrian monk named Gregor Mendel proposed that discrete units he called factors (later to be called *genes*) are passed down among family members to produce particular observable characteristics he called traits.

The scientific community didn't immediately act on Mendel's theory. Part of the problem was the novelty of the ideas. First, Mendel had presented his now famous garden pea experiments in a mathematical model. The math was simple enough, but biologists at that time were not used to interpreting experiments in mathematical terms.

There was a second reason for the gap between Mendel's work and the important work that followed from it. The very concept of cell division, crucial to Mendel's theory, had not yet been discovered. In fact, it was still unknown when Mendel died in 1884. But scientific progress soon changed that, leading to the identification and treatment of genetic diseases, including sickle cell disease.

One Hundred Years of Sickle Cell Disease Research and Treatment

Sickle cell disease has probably been in the world for thousands of years. There are African writings that described the symptoms of sickle cell and gave it names like *chwecheechwe*, *abututuo*, *nuidudui*, and *nwiiwii*. The first published reports of sickle cell disease in African medical literature were in the 1870s.

1910

More than one hundred years ago, the first well documented American case of sickle cell disease described was that of Walter Clement Noel, a first-year dental student at the Chicago College of Dental Surgery. Noel, who grew up in Grenada and moved to Chicago to attend dental school, was admitted to the Presbyterian Hospital in late 1904. He had leg ulcers, dizziness, and a breathing problem. Ernest E. Irons, a 27-year-old intern, obtained Noel's history and performed routine physical, blood, and urine examinations. Irons noticed that Noel's blood smear contained "many pear-shaped and elongated forms" and alerted his attending physician, James B. Herrick, to the unusual blood findings. Irons drew a rough sketch of these red blood cells in the hospital record. Herrick and Irons followed Noel over the next two-and-a-half years through several episodes of severe illness. Then Noel returned to Grenada to practice dentistry. He died nine years later at the age of 32 of pneumonia or acute chest syndrome. Herrick published the report "Peculiar elongated and sickle-shaped red blood corpuscles in a case of severe anemia" in the *Archives of Internal Medicine*, volume 6, pages 512–521, in 1910.

In that same year, Thomas Morgan, working at Columbia University, discovered from his research on fruit flies that genes are carried in chromosomes.

1917

V. E. Emmel reported in the *Archives of Internal Medicine* that the sickling observed by James Herrick occurred both in healthy individuals (with sickle trait) and in people who had anemia (sickle cell disease).

1927

Gillespie and Hahn demonstrated that it was a reduction in the oxygen content of the blood that led to the sickling of the red blood cells observed by Herrick. It was Hahn who first used the phrase "sickle cell trait" to describe those healthy individuals who had some sickling of red blood cells but no apparent anemia.

1944

Researchers at Rockefeller Institute in New York discovered that genes are made of deoxyribonucleic acid (DNA).

1948

Linus Pauling demonstrated, by comparing normal and sickle hemoglobin, that abnormal hemoglobin was the cause of sickle cell disease. In a paper titled "Sickle Cell Anemia, a Molecular Disease," published in *Science*, he explained how protein electrophoresis was used to show that sickle cell hemoglobin differed in structure from normal hemoglobin. This was the first time that the cause of a disease was linked to a change in protein structure.

1953

James Watson and Francis Crick, working at Cambridge University in England, carried this work a significant step further by uncovering the nature of the DNA molecule itself. The DNA, they noted, contains sugars, phosphates, and bases that are arranged in a spiral, complementary fashion, which they termed the "double helix." The DNA itself, in the nucleus of the cell, provides a blueprint for the making of protein in the cytoplasm.

1956

Vernon Ingram painstakingly arranged, without benefit of the automated gene sequencers we have today, in their exact order, the amino acids that make up hemoglobin. In this way Ingram showed for the first time that an amino acid called valine had replaced another amino acid called glutamic in the sixth position of the beta globin chain of hemoglobin. This very small change, as we all now know, had very great impact on the lives of people who suffer from it.

1960

Sydney Brenner, Matthew Meselson, and François Jacob discovered how information from the DNA in the nucleus is carried into the cytoplasm to make cells, identifying ribonucleic acid (RNA). RNA, coded by the DNA, carries the same configuration as the DNA into the cytoplasm and translates that message in the building of the cell's proteins.

1972

Congress passed the National Sickle Cell Anemia Control Act, and the NHLBI established Comprehensive Sickle Cell Centers.

1977

Walter Gilbert and Frederick Sanger developed new techniques for rapid DNA sequencing. This led to the identification of the mutation in the beta globin gene.

1980

The first statewide newborn screening program was implemented to detect sickle cell disease and trait at birth.

1984

The first 24-hour comprehensive sickle cell center opened at Grady Memorial Hospital in Atlanta, Georgia, offering specialized care outside the traditional emergency room.

Also in that year, the first sickle cell patient was cured by bone marrow transplant. By 2009, 276 bone marrow transplants had been done, with a 91%–97% survival rate and 7%–10% graft failure rate.

A new treatment option was also introduced in 1984. The medication hydroxyurea was found to increase fetal hemoglobin in sickle cell patients. This discovery has offered promising possibilities. In 1991, the Multicenter Study of Hydroxyurea in Sickle Cell Anemia (MSH) began. It was stopped early in 1995 because of proven benefits—reduced pain crises, reduced hospital admissions, and reduced need for blood transfusions. In 2003, a follow-up study reported that patients taking hydroxyurea have a prolonged life. And in 2008, a consensus statement from the NIH reported that more patients would benefit from hydroxyurea therapy.

1986

Penicillin Prophylaxis in Sickle Cell Disease, or PROPS, showed that prophylactic administration of penicillin to children from 6 months to age 6 prevents potentially fatal pneumococcal infection.

1987

The NIH held a consensus development conference on Newborn Screening for Sickle Cell Disease and Other Hemoglobinopathies and recommended that "every child should be screened for hemoglobinopathies to prevent the potentially fatal complications of sickle cell disease during infancy." In that year, 14 states were doing newborn screening for sickle cell; by 2002, 44 states did Hb screening, and by 2009 all 50 states were screening for hemoglobinopathies.

1995

Transfusion guidelines were first published. In surgical settings, simple transfusions to increase hemoglobin (Hb) levels to 10 g/dL are as good as or safer than aggressive transfusions to reduce sickle hemoglobin (Hb S) levels to below 30 percent. Researchers have found that transfusions to maintain a hematocrit of more than 36 percent do not reduce complications of pregnancy.

1997

The Stroke Prevention Trial in Sickle Cell Anemia (STOP) demonstrated that periodic transfusions could prevent first time stroke in susceptible children. Researchers have found that transcranial Doppler ultrasound (TCD) screening is effective in predicting which children are at highest risk for strokes. All sickle cell disease patients 24 months of age should be screened, and this screening should be repeated every 6–12 months during early childhood.

1997

Investigators inserted the human gene responsible for sickle cell disease into mice, thereby creating transgenic models of the human disease known as sickle cell mice. This breakthrough has led to important new developments..

1998

Doctors at the Aflac Cancer Center of Egleston Children's Hospital at Emory University in Atlanta performed the first unrelated donor cord blood stem transplant on Keone Penn, a 12-year-old with sickle cell anemia. He was cured of his sickle cell disease, but he had complications from the transplant.

2000

Pneumococcal conjugate vaccine (PCV), known as Prevnar, was released for immunization. By administering PCV, pneumococcal infections went from 1.7 infections per 100 person-years (1995–2000) to 0.5 infections per 100 person-years (2001–2002), which represents a 68% reduction. This has saved lives.

2003

The Human Genome Project was completed. Started in 1990, the US Human Genome Project, coordinated by the US Department of Energy and the National Institutes of Health, identified all the approximately 20,000–25,000 genes in human DNA and determined the sequences of the 3 billion chemical base pairs.

2005

The FDA approved Exjade (deferasirox), an oral iron chelator, for the treatment of iron overload.

2006

Senators Jim Talent, Charles Schumer, and Richard Burr provided support during African American Health Month by authoring a letter requesting funding in the FY07 Labor, Health and Human Services, and Education appropriations bill to create 40 treatment centers to provide medical treatment and education services for patients living with sickle cell disease. Several senators signed the letter by April 2006, requesting the funding to support the program.

2007

The National Athletic Trainers Association presented its consensus statement Sickle Cell and the Athlete, identifying 13 football player deaths, as well as numerous illnesses and deaths in basketball and distance running. Continuing from these findings, the 2008–09 NCAA Sports Medicine Handbook recommended excluding students with sickle cell disease from serial sprints and performance tests. The handbook recommended that athletes stop if they experience cramps or sudden weakness, or have trouble breathing. The NCAA recommended that athletes train over time but not push past endurance.

2008

Scientists at St. Jude's Research Hospital used a virus to correct the sickle gene in sickle cell mouse blood cells.

2009

June 19 was the First Sickle Cell Disease World Day at the United Nations, established to bring global awareness and focus on sickle cell disease.

Reversal on the stem cell research ban opened the way for new treatments. In December 2009, the New England Journal of Medicine reported that 10 adults with sickle cell disease received a partial bone marrow transplant with a 90% success rate.

2014
The TWiTCH trial (Transcranial Doppler with Transfusions Changing to Hydroxyurea) ended early, revealing that treatment with hydroxyurea is equal to regular blood transfusions in lowering brain blood flow noise in children at high risk for stroke.

New NIH evidence-based sickle cell guidelines are published at *www.nhlbi.nih.gov/health-pro/guidelines/sickle-cell-disease-guidelines*.

2015
Gene therapy breakthroughs—the modified stem cells from sickle cell patient bone marrow are able to make normal hemoglobin to a level of 20%.

2017
FDA approved Endari (L-glutamine oral powder), developed by Emmaus Life Sciences for use as a preventative in sickle cell patients five years of age and older.

"Gene Therapy in a Patient with Sickle Cell Disease," a report of the first successful case of using gene therapy in a patient with sickle cell disease in Paris, France, is published in the *New England Journal of Medicine*. Gene therapy that delivered an anti-sickling variant of hemoglobin in an autologous hematopoietic stem cell (HSC) transplant had relieved all the symptoms of severe sickle cell disease in a fifteen-year-old boy two years out from the procedure.

2018
The National Institutes of Health announced the launch of a new initiative to help speed the development of cures for sickle cell disease, a group of inherited blood disorders affecting at least 100,000 people in the United States and 20 million worldwide. The Cure Sickle Cell Initiative will take advantage of the latest genetic discoveries and technological advances to move the most promising genetic-based curative therapies safely into clinical trials within five to ten years.

Glossary

Acute chest syndrome—When sickled red blood cells block blood flow to the lungs. This can cause chest pain, shortness of breath, and cough. It is treated in the hospital with blood transfusions. It can be prevented with incentive spirometry or a blow bottle.

Amniocentesis—A test done by taking a small amount of fluid from the womb of a pregnant woman to determine if the baby has sickle cell disease or another genetic problem. This is usually performed when the pregnancy is 15–18 weeks along.

Anemia—A low red blood cell count. Anemia can be caused by many different events, including sickle cell disease.

Aplastic anemia or aplastic crisis—Decreased red blood cell count due to the bone marrow factory temporarily shutting down. The most common cause is a virus called Parvo B19.

Bone marrow—The blood factory inside of your big bones that makes red blood cells, white blood cells, and platelets.

Bone marrow transplant—A procedure that kills the existing bone marrow factory and plants donor (usually a matched brother or sister) marrow by transfusion. The bone marrow begins to make blood cells according to the genetic code of the donor. This has cured several sickle cell patients.

Carrier—One who inherits only one gene for a genetic problem like sickle cell. Usually there are no symptoms, and the carrier will never have the disease. Two carriers have a 25% risk of having a child with the disease.

Chorionic villus sampling (CVS)—This is a procedure to determine if a baby in the womb has a genetic disease like sickle cell. It is done when the pregnancy is 10–12 weeks along. A catheter or needle is used to get a sample of the placenta for testing.

Chromosome—The DNA code for all the parts of the human body. Each person has 46 individual chromosomes in cells, 23 donated from each parent. Chromosome 11 is where the sickle cell mutation occurs.

Complete blood count (CBC)—A blood test that gives clinicians information about how many red cells, white cells, and platelets a person has in their bloodstream.

Cord blood—This is the blood remaining in the umbilical cord and placenta after a baby is born and the cord is cut. This blood is rich in stem cells that can be saved and used in transplants.

Endari (L-glutamine)—L-glutamine oral powder is a new medication for sickle cell disease. It was approved by the FDA in 2017 and first entered the US market in 2018 under the brand name Endari. It works primarily by boosting the antioxidant properties of the red blood cell, helping the body fight oxidant damage and cut down on inflammation.

Erythrocytapheresis—Using a machine called a cell separator to separate the red blood cells, white blood cells, platelets, and plasma so that the red cells can be removed and the rest of the patient's blood be given back to them with new red blood cells that contain normal hemoglobin.

FARMS—An acronym to help you remember ways you can manage your sickle cell symptoms: **F**luids/Fever (drink plenty of liquids and manage fevers), **A**ir (get enough oxygen and be careful at high altitudes), **R**est (get plenty of sleep), **M**edication (e.g. penicillin, hydroxyurea, folic acid), and **S**ituations to avoid (e.g. stress, extreme temperatures, dehydration, drugs and alcohol).

Folic acid or folate—A B vitamin necessary for making new red blood cells. It also acts as a vasodilator, which allows your blood to flow more freely through small blood vessels, and it helps homocysteine level, which may reduce your risk of complications such as stroke, leg ulcers, and heart attack. Most sickle cell patients should take 1 mg a day. It is found in green, leafy vegetables, fruits, and whole grains.

Gallbladder—A pouch in the right upper abdomen under the liver. It stores bile to help digest fats in the diet.

Gallstones—Too much bilirubin from red blood cell breakdown can cause stones to form in the gallbladder. This can cause pain in the right upper abdomen, nausea, and indigestion when eating fatty foods. The gallbladder can be removed if it is full of stones.

Genes—These are the basic units of inheritance. They are located on chromosomes.

Gene therapy—Treatment that will change the genetic defect or the gene product (hemoglobin) in sickle cell disease. This is experimental at this time.

Hand-foot syndrome or dactylitis—Swelling and pain in the hands and feet, usually seen in six-month- to three-year-old sickle cell patients.

Hemoglobin—The protein substance inside the red blood cells that holds and releases oxygen. This is where the sickle mutation occurs.

Hemoglobin electrophoresis—The blood test that identifies the type of hemoglobins present in the red blood cells.

Hemoglobin AS—This is sickle cell trait, which results from the inheritance of a normal A hemoglobin gene and a sickle hemoglobin gene.

Hemoglobin S beta thalassemia—This is a type of sickle cell disease in which one inherits an S gene and a beta thalassemia gene from his or her parents. $S\beta^0$ thalassemia is more severe than $S\beta^+$ thalassemia.

Hemoglobin SC—A type of sickle cell disease in which one inherits an S gene and a C gene from the parents. This causes sickle cell complications, with increased eye and bone problems. Life expectancy is longer than with hemoglobin SS.

Hemoglobin SS—This is called sickle cell anemia and is the most common form of sickle cell disease.

Hemolysis—The breaking apart of red blood cells. Normal red cells last 120 days; sickled red blood cells last about fourteen days.

Hydroxyurea—The first medication for sickle cell disease that increases fetal hemoglobin. It reduces pain events by one half, the need for hospital admissions, and the need for blood transfusions—and it prolongs the lifespan.

Intravenous (IV)—A small plastic catheter placed in a vein to allow water, blood, or medication to enter the blood stream directly.

Jaundice—A yellow color in the white part (sclera) of the eye produced by increased bilirubin in the blood. Usually caused by increased red blood cell breakdown in sickle cell patients.

LOCATES—An acronym to help you remember how to record your pain: **L**ocation (where does it hurt?), **O**ther symptoms, **C**haracter (is the pain deep, burning?), **A**ggravating and alleviating things (what makes the pain worse or better?), **T**iming (when did it start?), **E**nvironment and effect (what was happening when the pain started, and how does it affect you?), and **S**everity.

Magnetic resonance imaging (MRI)—A large magnet-based device that painlessly creates images of the brain and other organs of the body

Pain episode or "crisis"—Pain in the bones and muscles where blood flow has been blocked by sickled red blood cells.

Portacath—An under-the-skin port that requires only a one-time needle stick that allows long-term painless access to sample venous blood, and/or to give IV fluids and medications.

Priapism—A prolonged painful erection of the penis from trapped sickled red blood cells.

Pulmonary hypertension—The condition in which the lungs' blood vessels are abnormally tight and raise the blood pressure there.

Reticulocyte count or "retics"—The count of brand new red blood cells just released from the bone marrow factory. It is the best indicator of how the bone marrow factory is producing red cells.

Sequestration—Blocked blood flow from sickled red blood cells in the spleen or liver. Blood can flow in, but it cannot flow out. This causes weakness, abdominal pain, and swelling of the liver or spleen.

Spleen—An organ in the left upper area of the stomach that helps filter germs from the blood stream.

Stroke—Blocked blood flow to an area of the brain that can cause weakness, numbness, trouble speaking, or trouble thinking.

Transcranial Doppler (TCD)—a special ultrasound device that uses painless sound waves to check for blocked blood flow in the brain. This test can identify children at greatest risk of having a stroke.

Bibliography

Adams, R. J., V. C. McKie, L. Hsu, et al. "Prevention of a first stroke by transfusions in children with sickle cell anemia and abnormal results on transcranial Doppler ultrasonography." *New England Journal of Medicine* 339, no. 1 (1998): 5–11.

Adeodu, O. O., T. Alimi, and A. D. Adekile. "A comprehensive study of the perception of sickle cell anemia by married Nigerian rural and urban women: Complications of sickle cell trait." *West African Journal of Medicine* 19, no. 1 (2000): 1–5.

Aldrich, T. K., S. K. Dhuper, W. S. Patwa, E. Makolo, S. M. Suzuka, S. A. Najeebi, S. Santhanakrishnan, R. L. Nagel, and M. E. Fabry. "Pulmonary entrapment of sickle cells: The role of regional alveolar hypoxia." *Journal of Applied Physiology* 80, no. 2 (1996): 531–39.

Alegre, M.-L., K. Gastadello, D. Abramovicz, P. Kinnaert, P. Vereerstraeten, L. DePauw, P. Vandenabeele, M. Moser, O. Leo, and M. Goldman. "Evidence that pentoxifylline reduces anti-CD3 monoclonal antibody-induced cytokine release syndrome." *Transplantation* 52, no. 4 (1991): 674–79.

Al-Salem, A. H., and S. Oaisruddin. "The significance of biliary sludge in children with sickle cell disease." *Pediatric Surgery International* 13, no. 1 (1998): 14–16.

Aluoch, J. R. "The presence of sickle cells in the peripheral blood film: Specificity and sensitivity of diagnosis of homozygous sickle cell disease in Kenya." *Tropical & Geographical Medicine* 47, no. 2 (1995): 89–91.

Aluoch, J. R. "Higher resistance to plasmodium falciparum infection in patients with homozygous sickle cell disease in western Kenya." *Tropical Medicine & International Health* 2, no. 6 (1997): 568–71.

American College of Physicians. 2008. "Summaries for patients: Pain and health care visits in patients with sickle cell disease." *Annals of Internal Medicine* 148, no. 2 (2008): 94–101.

American Medical Association. "Council report: Guidelines for handling parenteral antineoplastics." *Journal of the American Medical Association* 233, no. 11 (1985): 1590–92.

American Society of Hospital Pharmacists. "Technical assistance bulletin on handling cytotoxic and hazardous drugs." *American Journal of Hospital Pharmacy* 47, no. 3 (1990): 1033–49.

Angelkort, B. "Thrombozytenfunktion, plasmatische blutgerinnung und fibrinolyse bei chronisch arterieller verschlusskranheit." *Die Medizinische Welt* 30, no. 34 (1979): 1239–43.

Angelkort, B., N. Maurin, and K. Booteng. "Influence of pentoxifylline on erythrocyte deformability in peripheral occlusive disease." *Current Medical Research and Opinion* 6, no. 4 (1979): 255–58.

Armitage, J. O. "Bone Marrow Transplantation." In *Harrison's Principles of Internal Medicine, 14th ed.*, ed. A. S. Fauci, E. Braunwald, D. L. Kaspar, S. L. Hauser, D. L. Longo, J. L. Jameson, and J. Loscalzo, 724–30. New York: McGraw-Hill, 1998.

Arnold, S. D., M. Bhatia, J. Horan and L. Krishnamurti. "Haematopoietic stem cell transplantation for sickle cell disease—current practice and new approaches." *British Journal of Haematology* 174, no. 4 (2016): 515-525.

Assimadi, J. K., A. D. Gbadoe, and M. Nyadanu. "The impact on families of sickle cell disease in Togo." *Archives of Pediatrics & Adolescent Medicine* 7, no. 6 (2000): 615–620.

Ataga, K. I., and E. P. Orringer. "Renal abnormalities in sickle cell disease." *American Journal of Hematology* 63, no. 4 (2000): 205–11.

Baird, J. K., D. J. Fryauff, H. Basri, M. J. Bangs, B. Subianto, I. Wiady, B. Leksana, S. Masbar, T. L. Richie, T. R. Jones, E. Tjitra, S. Wignall, and S. L. Hoffman. "Primaquine for prophylaxis among nonimmune transmigrants in Irian Jaya, Indonesia." *American Journal of Tropical Medicine and Hygiene* 52, no. 6 (1995): 479–84.

Ballas, S. K. "The cost of health care for patients with sickle cell disease." *American Journal of Hematology* 84, no. 6 (2009): p. 320–22.

Ballas, S. K., and N. Mohandas. "Pathophysiology of vaso-occlusion." *Hematology/Oncology Clinics of North America* 10, no. 6 (1996): 1221–39.

Ballas, S. K., A. M. Zeidan, V. H. Duong, M. DeVeaux and M. M. Heeney. "The effect of iron chelation therapy on overall survival in sickle cell disease and beta-thalassemia: a systematic review." *American Journal of Hematology* 93, no. 7 (2018): 943-952.

Behrens, R. J., and T. C. Cymet. "Sickle cell disorders: Evaluation, treatment, and natural history." *Hospital Physician* 36, no. 9 (2000): 17–28.

Belgrave, F. Z., and S. D. Molock. "The role of depression in hospital admissions and emergency treatment of patients with sickle cell disease." *Journal of the National Medical Association* 83, no. 9 (1991): 777–81.

Bellet, P. S., K. A. Kalinyak, R. Shukla, M. J. Gelfand, D. L. Rucknagel. "Incentive spirometry to prevent acute pulmonary complications in sickle cell diseases." *New England Journal of Medicine* 333, no. 11 (1995): 699–703.

Benjamin, G. C. "Sickle cell anemia." In *The Cambridge World History of Human Disease*, ed. K. F. Kiple, 1006–07. Cambridge, UK: Cambridge University Press, 1993.

Benjamin, L. J., et al. *Guideline for the management of acute and chronic pain in sickle cell disease—American Pain Society clinical practice guidelines series, no. 1.* Glenview, IL: American Pain Society, 1999.

Beutler, E. "The sickle cell diseases and related disorders." In *Williams Hematology, 5th ed.*, ed. E. Beutler, et al., 616–54. New York: McGraw-Hill, 1995.

Beutler, E. "Disorders of hemoglobin." In *Harrison's Principles of Internal Medicine, 14th ed.*, ed. A. S. Fauci, E. Braunwald, D. L. Kaspar, S. L. Hauser, D. L. Longo, J. L. Jameson, and J. Loscalzo, 645–52. New York: McGraw-Hill, 1998.

Bitanga, E., and J. D. Rouillon. 1998. Influence of sickle cell trait on energy and abilities. *Pathologie Biologie (Paris)* 46(1): 46–52.

Bloom, M. *Understanding sickle cell disease*. Jackson, MS: University Press of Mississippi, 1999.

Boogaerts, M. A., S. Milbrain, P. Meerus, L. van Hove, and G. E. G. Verhoef. "In vitro modulation of normal human neutrophil function by pentoxifylline." *Blut* 61, no. 2–3 (1990): 60–65.

Brandow, A. M. and M. R. DeBaun. "Key components of pain management for children and adults with sickle cell disease." *Hematology/Oncology Clinics of North America* 32, no. 3 (2018): 535-550.

Brawley, O. W., et al. "National Institutes of Health consensus development conference statement: Hydroxyurea treatment for sickle cell disease." *Annals of Internal Medicine* 148, no. 12 (2008): 932–38.

Brewin, J., B. Kaya and S. Chakravorty. "How I manage sickle cell patients with high transcranial Doppler results." *British Journal of Haematology* 179, no. 3 (2017): 377-388.

Bruno, D., D. R. Wigfall, S. A. Zimmerman, P. M. Rosoff, and J. S. Wiener. "Genitourinary complications of sickle cell disease." *Journal of Urology* 166, no. 3 (2001): 803–11.

Bunn, H. F. Pathogenesis and treatment of sickle cell disease. *New England Journal of Medicine* 337, no. 11 (1997): 762–69.

Burlew, K., J. Telfair, L. Colangelo, and E. L. Wright. "Factors that influence adolescent adaptation to sickle cell disease." *Journal of Pediatric Psychology* 25, no. 5 (2000): 287–99.

Cao, A. "1993 William Allan Award address." *American Journal of Human Genetics* 54, no. 3 (1994): 397–402.

Cartwright, K. "Meningococcal carriage and disease." In *Meningococcal Disease*, ed. K. Cartwright, 115–46. Chichester, UK: John Wiley & Sons, 1995.

Castro, O., D. J. Brambilla, B. Thorington, et al. "The acute chest syndrome in sickle cell disease: Incidence and risk factors—The cooperative study of sickle cell disease." *Blood* 84, no. 2 (1994):643–49.

Centers for Disease Control and Prevention. *Health information for international travelers: HHS pub. no. 96–8280.* Washington, DC: US Department of Health and Human Services, 1996.

Centers for Disease Control and Prevention. "Mortality among children with sickle cell disease identified by newborn screening during 1990–1994—California, Illinois, and New York." *Morbidity and Mortality Weekly Report* 47, no. 9 (1998): 169–72.

Cepeda, M. L., F. H. Allen, N. J. Cepeda, and Y. M. Yang. "Physical growth, sexual maturation, body image, and sickle cell disease." *Journal of the National Medical Association* 92, no. 1 (2000): 10–14.

Chambers, J. B., D. A. Forsythe, S. L. Betrano, H. J. Iwinski, and D. E. Steflik. "Retrospective review of osteoarticular in a pediatric sickle cell age group." *Journal of Pediatric Orthopaedics* 20, no. 5 (2000): 682–85.

Chang, Y. P., M. Maier-Redelsperger, K. D. Smith, et al. "The relative importance of the X-linked FCP locus and beta-globin haplotypes in determining haemoglobin F levels: A study of SS patients homozygous for beta S haplotypes." *British Journal of Haematology* 96, no. 4 (1997): 806–14.

Chao, N. J., S. M. Schmidt, J. C. Niland, M. D. Amylon, A. C. Dagis, G. N. Long, A. P. Nadananee, R. S. Negron, M. R. O'Donnell, P. M. Parker, E. P. Smith, D. S. Snyder, A. S. Stein, R. M. Wong, K. G. Blume, and S. J. Forman. "Cyclosporine, methotrexate, and prednisone compared with cyclosporine and prednisone for prophylaxis of acute graft-vs-host disease." *New England Journal of Medicine* 329, no. 17 (1993): 1225–30.

Charache, S., F. B. Barton, R. D. Moore, M. L. Terrin, M. H. Steinberg, G. J. Dover, S. K. Ballas, R. P. McMahon, O. Castro, and E. P. Orringer. "Hydroxyurea and sickle cell anemia: Clinical utility of a myelosuppressive 'switching' agent—The multicenter study of hydroxyurea in sickle cell anemia." *Medicine* 75, no. 6 (1996): 300–326.

Charache, S., G. J. Dover, R. D. Moore, S. Eckert, S. K. Ballas, M. Koshy, P. F. Millner, E. P. Orringer, G. Phillips Jr., O. S. Platt, and G. U. Thomas. "Hydroxyurea: Effects on hemoglobin F production in patients with sickle cell anemia." *Blood* 79, no. 10 (1992): 2555–65.

Charache, S., M. L. Terrin, R. D. Moore, et al. "Effect of hydroxyurea on the frequency of painful crises in sickle cell anemia." *New England Journal of Medicine* 332, no. 20 (1995): 1317–22.

Chinegwundoh, F., and K. A. Anie. "Treatments for priapism in boys and men with sickle cell disease." *Cochrane Database of Systematic Reviews* 18, no. 4 (2004): CD004198.

Cipolotti, R., M. F. Caskey, et al. "Childhood and adolescent growth of patients with sickle cell disease in Aracaju, Sergipe, north-east Brazil." *Annals of Tropical Paediatrics* 20, no. 2 (2000): 109–13.

Clark, C. "Gene therapy: A promising strategy for sickle cell anemia." *Blood Weekly* June 22 (1998): 13.

Clift, R. A., C. D. Bucker, F. R. Appelbaum, G. Schoch, F. B. Peterson, W. I. Bensinger, W. J. Senders, R. M. Sullivan, R. Storb, and J. Singer. "Allogeneic marrow transplantation during untreated first relapse of acute myeloid leukemia." *Journal of Clinical Oncology* 10, no. 11 (1992): 1723–29.

Clinical Oncological Society of Australia. "Guidelines and recommendations for safe handling of antineoplastic agents." *Medical Journal of Australia* 1 (1983): 426–28.

Coates, T. D. and J. C. Wood. "How we manage iron overload in sickle cell patients." *British Journal of Haematology* 177, no. 5 (2017): 703-716.

Consensus Conference. "Newborn screening for sickle cell disease and other hemoglobinopathies." *Journal of the American Medical Association* 258, no. 9 (1987): 1205–09.

Crystal, R. G. "Transfer of genes to humans: Early lessons and obstacles to success." *Science* 270, no. 5235 (1995): 404–10.

Davies, S. M., X. O. Shu, B. R. Blazar, A. H. Filipovich, J. H. Kersey, W. Krivit, J. McCullough, W. J. Miller, N. K. C. Ramsay, M. Segall, J. E. Wagner, D. J. Weisdorf, and P. B. McGlave. "Unrelated donor bone marrow transplantation: Influence of HLA A and B incompatibility on outcome." *Blood* 86, no. 4 (1995): 1636–42.

Davis, B. A., S. Allard, A. Qureshi, J. B. Porter, S. Pancham, N. Win, G. Cho and K. Ryan (2017). "Guidelines on red cell transfusion in sickle cell disease. Part I: Principles and laboratory aspects." *British Journal of Haematology* 176, no. 2 (2017): 179-191.

Davis, B. A., S. Allard, A. Qureshi, J. B. Porter, S. Pancham, N. Win, G. Cho and K. Ryan. "Guidelines on red cell transfusion in sickle cell disease. Part II: Indications for transfusion." *British Journal of Haematology* 176, no. 2 (2017): 192-209.

Davis, H., R. M. Moore Jr., and P. J. Gergen. "Cost of hospitalizations associated with sickle cell disease in the United States." *Public Health Reports* 112, no. 1 (1997): 40–43.

DeBaun, M. R. and F. J. Kirkham. "Central nervous system complications and management in sickle cell disease." *Blood* 127, no. 7 (2016): 829-838.

Derchi, G., G. L. Forni, F. Formisano, M. D. Cappellini, R. Galanello, G. D'Ascola, P. Bina, C. Magnano, and M. Lamagna. "Efficacy and safety of sildenafil in the treatment of severe pulmonary hypertension in patients with hemoglobinopathies." *Haematologica* 90, no. 4 (2005): 452–58.

Desai, P. C. and K. I. Ataga. "The acute chest syndrome of sickle cell disease." *Expert Opinion on Pharmacotherapy* 14, no. 8 (2013): 991-999.

Dormandy, J., G. B. Nash, T. Loosemore, and P. R. Thomas. "Effects of acute trental on white cell rheology in patients with critical leg ischemia." In *Pentoxifylline and Analogues: Effects on Leukocyte Function*, ed. J. Hakim, G. L. Mandell, and W. J. Novick Jr., 203–05. Basel, Switzerland: S. Karger, 1990.

Eckman, J. R. "Techniques for blood administration in sickle cell patients." *Seminars in Hematology* 38, no. 1, suppl. 1 (2001): 23–29.

Eckman, J. R., and A. F. Platt. *Problem Oriented Management of Sickle Cell Syndromes, 4th ed: NIH pub. no. 02-2117*. Bethesda, MD: National Institutes of Health, National Heart, Lung, and Blood Center, 1991, 2002.

Egrie, J. C., T. W. Strickland, J. Lane, K. Aoki, A. M. Cohen, R. Smalling, G. Trail, F. K. Lin, J. K. Browne, and D. K. Hines. "Characterization and biological effects of recombinant human erythropoietin." *Immunobiology* 172, no. 3–5 (1986): 213–24.

Ehlers, K. H., P. J. Giardina, M. L. Lesser, M. A. Engle, and M. W. Hilgartner. "Prolonged survival in patients with beta-thalassemia treated with deferoxamine." *Journal of Pediatrics* 118, no. 4 (1991): 540–45.

Embury, S. H., J. F. Garcia, N. Mohandas, R. Pennathur-Das, and M. R. Clark. "Effects of oxygen inhalation on endogenous erythropoietin kinetics, erythropoiesis, and properties of blood cells in sickle-cell anemia." *New England Journal of Medicine* 311, no. 5 (1984): 291–95.

Embury, S. H., R. P. Hebbel, and N. Mohandas, eds. *Sickle Cell Diseases: Basic Principles and Clinical Practice.* Hagerstown, MD: Lippincott-Raven, 1994.

Eschbach, J. W., J. C. Egrie, M. R. Downing, J. K. Browne, and J. W. Adamson. "Correction of the anemia of end-stage renal disease with recombinant human erythropoietin." *New England Journal of Medicine* 316, no. 2 (1987): 73–78.

Eschbach, J. W., J. C. Egrie, M. R. Downing, J. K. Browne, and J. W. Adamson. "The use of recombinant human erythropoietin (r-HuEPO): Effect in end-stage renal disease (ESRD)." In *Prevention of Chronic Uremia*, ed. E. A. Friedman, M. Boyer, N. G. DeSanto, and C. Giordano, 148–55. Philadelphia: Field and Wood Inc., 1989.

Fedson, D. S., and D. M. Musher. "Pneumococcal vaccine." In *Vaccines, 2nd ed.*, ed. S. A. Plotkin and E. A. Mortimer Jr., 517. Philadelphia: Saunders, 1994.

Ferrari, E., M. Fioravanti, A. L. Patti, and C. Viola. "Effects of long-term treatment (four years) with pentoxifylline on hemorrheological changes and vascular complications in diabetic patients." *Pharmatherapeutica* 5 , no. 1 (1987): 26–39.

Field, J. J., J. E. Knight-Perry, and M. R. Debaun. "Acute pain in children and adults with sickle cell disease: Management in the absence of evidence-based guidelines." *Current Opinion in Hematology* 16, no. 3 (2009): 173–78.

Firth, P. G., and R. A. Peterfreund. "Management of multiple intracranial aneurysms: Neuroanesthetic considerations of sickle cell disease." *Journal of Neurosurgical Anesthesiology* 12, no. 4 (2000): 366–71.

Fitzgerald, R. K., and A. Johnson. 2001. Pulse oximetry in sickle cell anemia. *Critical Care Medicine* 29(9): 1803–06.

Fitzhugh, C. D., D. R. Wigfall, and R. E. Ware. "Enalapril and hydroxyurea therapy for children with sickle nephropathy." *Pediatric Blood & Cancer* 45, no. 7 (2005): 982–85.

Fleming, D. R., N. K. Rayens, and J. Garrison. "Impact of obesity on allogeneic stem cell transplant patients: A matched case-controlled study." *American Journal of Medicine* 102, no. 3 (1997): 265–68.

Frasch, C. E. "Meningococcal vaccines: Past, present, and future." In *Meningococcal Disease*, ed. K. Cartwright, 35–70. Chichester, UK: John Wiley & Sons, 1995.

Gaston, M. H, J. L. Verter, G. Woods, et al. "Prophylaxis with oral penicillin in children with sickle cell anemia: A randomized trial." *New England Journal of Medicine* 314, no. 25 (1986): 1593–99.

Gill, F. M., L. A. Sleeper, S. J. Weiner, et al. "Clinical events in the first decade in a cohort of infants with sickle cell disease—The cooperative study of sickle cell disease." *Blood* 86, no. 2 (1995): 776–83.

Glickman, E., M. M. Horowitz, R. E. Chanopin, J. M. Hows, A. Bacigalapo, J. L. Biggs, B. M. Camitta, R. P. Gale, L. C. Gordon-Smith, A. M. Marmont, T. Masuoka, N. K. C. Ramsay, A. Rima, C. Rozman, K. A. Sabocinski, B. Speck, and M. M. Bortin. "Bone marrow transplantation for severe aplastic anemia: Influence of conditioning and severe graft-vs-host disease prophylaxis regimens on outcome." *Blood* 79, no. 1 (1992): 269–75.

Godeau, B., F. Galacteros, A. Schaeffer, F. Morinet, D. Bachir, J. Rosa, and J. L. Portos. "Aplastic crisis due to extensive bone marrow necrosis and human parvovirus infection in sickle cell disease." *American Journal of Medicine* 91, no. 5 (1991): 557–58.

Goldstein, M. *The Nature of Animal Healing*. New York: Alfred A Knopf, 1999.

Graber, S. E., and S. B. Krantz. "Erythropoietin and the control of red cell production." *Annual Review of Medicine* 29 (1978): 51–58.

Grant, M. M., K. M. Gill, M. Y. Floyd, and M. Abrams. "Depression and functioning in relation to health care use in sickle cell disease." *Annals of Behavioral Medicine* 22, no. 2 (2000): 149–57.

Gucalp, R., and J. Dutcher. "Oncologic Emergencies." In *Harrison's Principles of Internal Medicine, 14th ed.*, ed. A. S. Fauci, E. Braunwald, D. L. Kaspar, S. L. Hauser, D. L. Longo, J. L. Jameson, and J. Loscalzo, 627–34. New York: McGraw-Hill, 1998.

Guilcher, G. M. T., T. H. Truong, S. L. Saraf, J. J. Joseph, D. Rondelli and M. M. Hsieh. "Curative therapies: allogeneic hematopoietic cell transplantation from matched related donors using myeloablative, reduced intensity, and nonmyeloablative conditioning in sickle cell disease." *Seminars in Hematology* 55, no. 2 (2018): 87-93.

Hassell, K. L., J. R. Eckman, and P. A. Lane. "Acute multiorgan failure syndrome: A potentially catastrophic complication of severe sickle cell pain episodes." *American Journal of Medicine* 96, no. 2 (1994): 155–62.

Hassell, K. L., B. Pace, W. Wang, R. Kulkarni, C. S. Johnson, J. Eckman, P. A. Lane, W. G. Woods, and American Society of Pediatric Hematology/Oncology. "Sickle cell disease summit: From clinical and research disparity to action." *American Journal of Hematology* 84, no. 1 (2009): 39–45.

Hillman, R. S. "Iron deficiency and other hypoproliferative anemias." In *Harrison's Principles of Internal Medicine, 14th ed.*, ed. A. S. Fauci, E. Braunwald, D. L. Kaspar, S. L. Hauser, D. L. Longo, J. L. Jameson, and J. Loscalzo, 638–45. New York: McGraw-Hill, 1998.

Hiruma, H., C. T. Noguchi, N. Uyesaka, S. Hasegawa, E. J. Blanchette-Mackie, A. N. Schecter, and G. P. Rodgers. "Sickle cell rheology is determined by polymer fraction—Not cell morphology." *American Journal of Hematology* 48, no. 1 (1995): 19–28.

Howard, J. "Sickle cell disease: when and how to transfuse." *Hematology—The Education Program of the American Society of Hematology* 2016, no. 1 (2016): 625-631.

Huang, A. W. and O. Muneyyirci-Delale. "Reproductive endocrine issues in men with sickle cell anemia." *Andrology* 5, no. 4 (2017): 679-690.

Human Genome Program. "Gene therapy." In *Human Genome Project Information*. Oak Ridge, TN: US Department of Energy, Office of Biological and Environmental Research, 2008.

Ibidapo, M. O., and O. O. Akinyaju. "Acute sickle cell syndromes in Nigerian adults." *Clinical and Laboratory Haematology* 22, no. 3 (2000): 151–55.

Israel, R. A., H. M. Rosenberg, and L. R. Curtin. "Analytical potential for multiple cause-of death data." *American Journal of Epidemiology* 124, no. 2 (1986): 161–79.

Itoh, T., S. Chien, and S. Usami. "Effects of hemoglobin concentration on individual sickle cells after deoxygenation." *Blood* 85, no. 8 (1995): 2245–53.

Jackson, B., R. Fasano and J. Roback. "Current evidence for the use of prophylactic transfusion to treat sickle cell disease during pregnancy." *Transfusion Medicine Reviews* 32, no. 4 (2018): 220-224.

Jean-Baptiste, G. A., and K. Leuleer. "Osteoarticular disorders of hematological origin." *Baillière's Best Practice & Research Clinical Rheumatology* 14, no. 2 (2000): 307–23.

Jim, R. T. S. "New therapy for microangiopathic hemolytic anemia caused by cardiac valve prosthesis: A case report." *Hawaii Medical Journal* 47, no. 6 (1988): 285.

Johns Hopkins University, "Half-match bone marrow transplants wipe out sickle cell disease in selected patients," news release, September 20, 2012, https://www.hopkinsmedicine.org/news/media/releases/half_match_bone_marrow_transplants_wipe_out_sickle_cell_disease_in_selected_patients.

Johnson, C., ed. "Sickle cell disease: Special issue." *Hematology/ Oncology Clinics of North America* 19, no. 5 (2005): 771–996.

Jones, R. B., R. Frank, and T. Mass. "Safe handling of chemotherapeutic agents: A report from the Mount Sinai Medical Center." *CA: A Cancer Journal for Clinicians* 33, no. 5 (1983): 258–63.

Kachmaryk, M. M., S. N. Trimble, and R. G. Gieser. "Cilioretinal artery occlusion in sickle cell trait." *Retina* 15, no. 6 (1995): 501–04.

Kark, J. A., D. M. Posey, H. R. Schumacher, and C. J. Ruehle. "Sickle-cell trait as a risk factor for sudden death in physical training." *New England Journal of Medicine* 317, no. 13 (1987): 781–86.

Kelly, S., K. Quirolo, A. Marsh, L. Neumayr, A. Garcia and B. Custer. "Erythrocytapheresis for chronic transfusion therapy in sickle cell disease: Survey of current practices and review of the literature." *Transfusion* 56, no. 11 (2016): 2877-2888.

Kerle, K. K., and K. D. Nishimura. "Exertional collapse and sudden death associated with sickle cell trait." *American Family Physician* 54, no. 1 (1996): 237–40.

King, A. A., D. A. White, R. C. McKinstry, M. Noetzel, and M. R. DeBaun. "A pilot randomized education rehabilitation trial is feasible in sickle cell and strokes." *Neurology* 68, no. 23 (2007): 2008–11.

Kinney, T. R., R. W. Helms, E. E. O'Branski, K. Ohen-Frempong, W. Wang, C. Daeschner, E. Vichinsky, R. Redding-Lallinger, B. Gee, O. S. Platt, and R. E. Ware. "Safety of hydroxyurea in children with sickle cell anemia: Results of the HUG-KIDS study, a phase I/II trial—Pediatric Hydroxyurea Group." *Blood* 94, no. 5 (1999): 1550–54.

Krause, P. J., K. G. Maderazo, J. Contrino, L. Eisenfeld, V. C. Herson, N. Greca, P. Bannon, and D. L. Kreutzer. "Modulation of neonatal neutrophil function by pentoxifylline." *Pediatric Research* 29, no. 2 (1991): 123–27.

Krishnamurti, L. "Hematopoietic cell transplantation: A curative option for sickle cell disease." *Journal of Pediatric Hematology/Oncology* 24, no. 8 (2007): 569–75.

Ladwig, P., and H. Murray. "Sickle cell disease in pregnancy." *Australian and New Zealand Journal of Obstetrics and Gynaecology* 40, no. 1 (2000): 97–100.

Lanzkron, S., C. Haywood Jr., J. B. Segal, and G. J. Dover. "Hospitalization rates and costs of care of patients with sickle-cell anemia in the state of Maryland in the era of hydroxyurea." *American Journal of Hematology* 81, no. 12 (2006): 927–32.

Leiken, S. L., D. Gallagher, T. R. Kinney, et al. "Mortality in children and adolescents with sickle cell disease—The cooperative study of sickle cell disease." *Pediatrics* 84, no. 3 (1989): 500–508.

Lell, B., J. May, and R. J. Schmidt. "The role of red blood cell polymorphism in resistance and susceptibility to malaria." *Clinical Infectious Diseases* 28, no. 4 (1999): 794–99.

Leonhardt, H., and H.-G. Grigoleit. "Effects of pentoxifylline on red blood cell deformability and blood viscosity under hyperosmolar conditions." *Naunyn-Schniedeberg's Archives of Pharmacology* 299, no. 2 (1977): 197–200.

Lorey, F. W., J. Arnopp, and G. Cunningham. "Distribution of hemoglobinopathy variants by ethnicity in a multiethnic state." *Genetic Epidemiology* 13, no. 5 (1996) : 501–512.

Lorey, F. W., G. Cunningham, F. Shafer, B. Lubin, and E. Vichinsky. "Universal screening for hemoglobinopathies using high-performance liquid chromatography: Clinical results of 2.2 million screens." *European Journal of Human Genetics* 2, no. 4 (1994): 262–71.

Lucarelli, G., M. Galimberti, P. Polchi, E. Angelucci, D. Barancianci, C. Giardini, P. Politi, S. M. Durazzi, P. Muretto, and F. Albertini. "Bone marrow transplantation in patients with thalassemia." *New England Journal of Medicine* 322, no. 7 (1990): 417–21.

Lundin, A. P., M. J. H. Akerman, and R. M. Chester. "Exercise in hemodialysis patients after treatment with recombinant human erythropoietin". *Nephron* 58, no. 3 (1991): 315–19.

Machado, R. F., S. Martyr, G. J. Kato, R. J. Barst, A. Anthi, M. R. Robinson, L. Hunter, W. Coles, J. Nichols, C. Hunter, V. Sachdev, O. Castro, and M. T. Gladwin. "Sildenafil therapy in patients with sickle cell disease and pulmonary hypertension." *British Journal of Haematology* 130, no. 3 (2005): 445–53.

Malinowski, A. K., N. Shehata, R. D'Souza, K. H. Kuo, R. Ward, P. S. Shah and K. Murphy. "Prophylactic transfusion for pregnant women with sickle cell disease: a Systematic review and meta-analysis." *Blood* 126, no. 21 (2015): 2424-2435; quiz 2437.

Manci, E. A., D. E. Culberson, Y. M. Yang, T. M. Gardner, R. Powell, J. Haynes Jr., A. K. Shah, and V. N. Mankad. "Investigators of the cooperative study of sickle cell disease—Causes of death in sickle cell disease: An autopsy study." *British Journal of Haematology* 123, no. 2 (2003): 359–65.

Marshall, E. "Gene therapy's growing pains." *Science* 269, no. 5227 (1995): 1050–55.

Marti-Carvajal, A. J., I. Sola and L. H. Agreda-Perez. "Treatment for avascular necrosis of bone in people with sickle cell disease." *Cochrane Database of Systematic Reviews* 8 (2016): CD004344.

Medical Economics. *Physicians' Desk Reference, 53rd ed.* Montvale, NJ: Medical Economics Inc., 1999.

Meshikhes, A.-W. N., S. A. al-Dhurais, A. al-Jama, et al. "Laparoscopic cholecystectomy in patients with sickle cell disease." *Journal of the Royal College of Surgeons of Edinburgh* 40, no. 6 (1995): 383–85.

Michlitsch, J. G., and M. C. Walters. "Recent advances in bone marrow transplantation in hemoglobinopathies." *Current Molecular Medicine* 8, no. 7 (2008): 675–89.

Minniti, C. P. and G. J. Kato. "Critical reviews: how we treat sickle cell patients with leg ulcers." *American Journal of Hematology* 91, no. 1 (2016): 22-30.

Modell, B. and Darlison, M. "Global Epidemiology Of Haemoglobin Disorders And Derived Service Indicators." *Bulletin of the World Health Organization* 86, no. 6 (2008): 480–487.

Mohan, J. S., J. E. Vigilance, J. M. Marshall, I. R. Hambleton, H. L. Reid, and G. R. Serjeany. "Abnormal venous function in patients with homozygous sickle cell (SS) disease and chronic leg ulcers." *Clinical Science (Colchester)* 98, no. 6 (2000): 667–72.

Morris, C. R., G. J. Kato, M. Poljakovic, X. Wang, W. C. Blackwelder, V. Sachdev, S. L. Hazen, E. P. Vichinsky, S. M. Morris Jr., and M. T. Gladwin. "Dysregulated arginine metabolism, hemolysis-associated pulmonary hypertension, and mortality in sickle cell disease." *Journal of the American Medical Association* 294, no. 1 (2005): 81–90.

Morris, C. R. "Asthma management: Reinventing the wheel in sickle cell disease." *American Journal of Hematology* 84, no. 4 (2009): 234–41.

Müller, R. "Hemorheology and peripheral vascular disease: A new therapeutic approach." *Journal of Medicine* 12, no. 4 (1981): 209–35.

Musher, D. M. "Pneumococcal Infections." In *Harrison's Principles of Internal Medicine, 14th ed.*, ed. A. S. Fauci, E. Braunwald, D. L. Kaspar, S. L. Hauser, D. L. Longo, J. L. Jameson, and J. Loscalzo, 869–75. New York: McGraw-Hill, 1998.

Nagel, R. L., and H. M. Ranney. 1990. Genetic epidemiology of structural mutations of the beta-globin gene. *Seminars in Hematology* 27(4): 342–59.

National Center for Biotechnology Information. "Hemoglobin—Beta locus; HBB." *Online Mendelian inheritance in man (OMIM). MIM no. 141900.* Baltimore, MD: The Johns Hopkins University, 1998. Available at: omim.org/entry/141900.

National Heart, Lung, and Blood Institute. *Collection and Storage of Umbilical Cord Stem Cells for Treatment of Sickle Cell Disease.* Bethesda, MD: National Institutes of Health, 2010.

National Human Genome Research Institute. *Learning About Sickle Cell Disease.* Bethesda, MD: National Institutes of Health, 2010.

National Institutes of Mental Health. *Recommendations for the Safe Handling of Parenteral Antineoplastic Drugs: NIH pub. no. 83-2621.* Washington, DC: US Department of Health and Human Services, 1983.

National Study Commission on Cytotoxic Exposure. *Recommendations for Handling Cytotoxic Agents.* Boston: Massachusetts College of Pharmacy and Allied Health Sciences, 1987.

NBC News, "Partial-match transplants ease the grinding pain of sickle cell disease," January 19, 2019, https://www.nbcnews.com/health/kids-health/less-perfect-still-good-partial-match-transplants-ease-pain-sickle-n958586.

Neonato, M. G., M. Guillod-Batalle, P. Beauvais, P. Beguei P, et al. "Acute clinical events in 299 homozygous sickle cell patients living in France—French study group on sickle cell disease." *European Journal of Haematology* 65, no 3 (2000): 155–64.

New York Newsday. "Briefs." December 1, 1999. A38.

Newborn Screening Committee, The Council of Regional Networks for Genetic Services (CORN). *National Newborn Screening Report—1993.* Atlanta: CORN, 1998.

Niihara Y., S. T. Miller, J. Kanter, S. Lanzkron, W. R. Smith, L. L. Hsu, V. R. Gordeuk, K. Viswanathan, S. Sarnaik, I. Osunkwo, E. Guillaume, S. Sadanandan, L. Sieger, J. L. Lasky, E. H. Panosyan, O. A. Blake, T. N. New, R. Bellevue, L. T. Tran, R. L. Razon, C. W. Stark, L. D. Neumayr, E. P. Vichinsky, et al. "A Phase 3 Trial of l-Glutamine in Sickle Cell Disease." *New England Journal of Medicine* 379, no. 3 (2018): 226-235.

Nietert, P. J., M. R. Abboud, M. D. Silverstein, and S. M. Jackson. "Bone marrow transplantation versus periodic prophylactic blood transfusion in sickle cell patients at high risk of ischemic stroke: A decision analysis." *Blood* 95, no. 10 (2000): 3057–64.

Nissenson, A. R., S. D. Nimer, and D. L. Wolcott. "Recombinant human erythropoietin and renal anemia: Molecular biology, clinical efficacy, and nervous system effects." *Annals of Internal Medicine* 114, no. 5 (1991): 402–16.

Norris, W. E. "Acute hepatic sequestration in sickle cell disease." *Journal of the American Medical Association* 96, no. 9 (2004): 1235–39.

Nwadiaro, H. C., B. T. Ugwu, and J. N. Legbo. "Chronic osteomyelitis in patients with sickle cell disease." *East African Medical Journal* 77, no. 1 (2000): 23–26.

Occupational Safety and Health Administration. "Controlling occupational exposure to hazardous drugs: OSHA work practice guidelines." *American Journal of Health-System Pharmacy* 53, no. 14 (1996): 1669–85.

Office of Science Policy. 2009. "About Recombinant DNA Advisory Committee (RAC)." In *Office of Biotechnology Activities*. Bethesda, MD: National Institutes of Health.

Ogandi, S. O., and F. Onwe. "A pilot survey comparing the level of sickle cell disease knowledge in a university of south Texas and a university in Enugu, Enugu state, Nigeria, West Africa." *Ethnicity and Disease* 10, no. 2 (2000): 232–36.

Ohene-Frempong, K. "Indications for red cell transfusion in sickle cell disease." *Seminars in Hematology* 38, no. 1, suppl. 1 (2001): 5–13.

Ohene-Frempong, K., S. J. Weiner, L. A. Sleeper, et al. "Cerebrovascular accidents in sickle cell disease: Rates and risk factors." *Blood* 91, no. 1 (1998): 288–94.

Osunkwo, I. "An update on the recent literature on sickle cell bone disease." *Current Opinion in Endocrinology, Diabetes, and Obesity* 20, no. 6 (2013): 539-546.

Oyesiku, N. M., J. R. Eckman, D. L. Barrow, S. C. Tindall, and A. R. Colohan. "Intracranial aneurysms in sickle cell anemia: Clinical features and pathogenesis." *Journal of Neurosurgery* 75, no. 3 (1991): 356–63.

Pace, Betty. "Gene Therapy for Sickle Cell Disease" in *Hope and Destiny*, fourth edition by Allan Platt, James Eckman, and Lewis L. Hsu (Chicago: Hilton Publishing, 2016), 165–173.

Paciocco, G., F. J. Martinez, E. Bossone, E. Pielsticker, B. Gillespie, and M. Rubenfire. "Oxygen desaturation on the six-minute walk test and mortality in untreated primary pulmonary hypertension." *European Respiratory Journal* 17, no. 4 (2001): 647–52.

Pack-Mabien, A., and J. Haynes Jr. "A primary care provider's guide to preventive and acute care management of adults and children with sickle cell disease." *Journal of the American Academy of Nurse Practitioners* 21, no. 5 (2009): 250–57.

Platt, O. S., D. J. Brambilla, W. F. Rosse, et al. "Mortality in sickle cell disease: Life expectancy and risk factors for early death." *New England Journal of Medicine* 330, no. 23 (1994): 1639–44.

Platt, O. S., B. D. Thorington, D. J. Brambilla, et al. "Pain in sickle cell disease—Rates and risk factors." *New England Journal of Medicine* 325, no. 1 (1991): 11–16.

Porter, J. B. "Concepts and goals in the management of transfusional iron overload." *American Journal of Hematology* 82, suppl. 12 (2007): 1136–39.

Powars, D., and A. Hiti. "Sickle cell anemia: Beta s gene cluster haplotypes as genetic markers for severe disease expression." *American Journal of Diseases of Children* 147, no. 11 (1993): 1197–1202.

Prabhakar, H. *Improving the Quality of Care for Sickle Cell Disease for Patients and Providers in the United States: A Review of General Considerations and Observations for Improving Health Systems Management of Sickle Cell Disease.* Baltimore, MD: The Johns Hopkins University, 2009.

Rahimy, M. C., A. Gangboa, R. Adjou, C. Deguenon, S. Goussanou, and E. Ahihonou. "Effect of active management on pregnancy outcome in sickle cell disease in an African setting." *Blood* 96, no. 5 (2000): 1685–89.

Reed, W., and E. P. Vichinsky. "Transfusion therapy: A coming-of-age treatment for patients with sickle cell disease." *Journal of Pediatric Hematology/Oncology* 23, no. 4 (2001): 197–202.

Rees, D. C., S. Robinson and J. Howard. "How I manage red cell transfusions in patients with sickle cell disease." *British Journal of Haematology* 180, no. 4 (2018): 607-617.

Ribeil, J. A., S. Hacein-Bey-Abina, E. Payen, A. Magnani, M. Semeraro, E. Magrin, L. Caccavelli, B. Neven, P. Bourget, W. El Nemer, P. Bartolucci, L. Weber, H. Puy, J. F. Meritet, D. Grevent, Y. Beuzard, S. Chrétien, T. Lefebvre, R. W. Ross, O. Negre, G. Veres, L. Sandler, S. Soni, M. de Montalembert, S. Blanche, P. Leboulch, M. Cavazzana. "Gene Therapy in a Patient with Sickle Cell Disease." *New England Journal of Medicine* 376, no. 9 (2017):848-855.

Sacerdote, A. "Treatment of homozygous sickle cell disease with pentoxifylline." *Journal of the National Medical Association* 91, no. 9 (1999): 466–70.

Sacerdote, A., and A. Bishnoi. "Enhanced reduction of proteinuria in diabetics with triple therapy: Pentoxifylline, protein restriction, and angiotensin converting enzyme inhibitors." *Diabetes* 38 supp (1989): 158A.

Sacerdote, A., and A. Bishnoi. "Triple therapy for proteinuria in diabetics; Pentoxifylline, protein restriction, and angiotensin converting enzyme inhibitors." *Clinical Research* 37 (1989): 860A.

Sacerdote, A., and M. Rodriguez. "Treatment of homozygous SS disease with pentoxifylline." *Clinical Research* 42, no. 2 (1994): 239A.

Schmetterer, L., D. Kemmler, H. Breitenender, C. Alschinger, R. Koppensteiner, F. Lexer, A. F. Fercher, H. Eichler, and M. Wolgt. "A randomized, placebo-controlled, double-blind crossover of the effect of pentoxifylline on ocular fundus pulsations." *American Journal of Opthalmology* 121, no. 2 (1996): 169–76.

Schubert, T. T. "Hepatobiliary system in sickle cell disease." *Gastroenterology* 90, no. 6 (1986): 2013.

Schubolz, R., and O. Mufellner. "The effect of pentoxifylline on erythrocyte deformability and phosphatide fatty acid distribution in the erythrocyte membrane." *Current Medical Research and Opinion* 4, no. 9 (1977): 609–17.

Segal, M. "New hope for children with sickle cell disease." *FDA Consumer* 23, no. 2(1989): 14–19.

Serjeant, G. R. "Sickle cell disease." *Lancet* 350, no. 9079 (1997): 725–30.

Shah, R., C. Taborda and S. Chawla. "Acute and chronic hepatobiliary manifestations of sickle cell disease: a review." *World Journal of Gastrointestinal Pathophysiolgy* 8, no. 3 (2017): 108-116.

Shanks, G. D. "Malaria prevention and prophylaxis." In *Ballière's Clinical Infectious Diseases, Vol. 2*, ed. G. Pasvol, 331–49. London, UK: Ballière Tindall, 1995.

Shapiro, E. D., A. T. Berg, R. Austrian, D. Schroeder, V. Parcells, A. Margolis, R. K. Adair, and J. D. Clemens. "The protective efficacy of polyvalent pneumococcal polysaccharide vaccine." *New England Journal of Medicine* 325, no. 21 (1991): 1453–60.

Sickle Cell Disease Guideline Panel. *Sickle Cell Disease: Screening, Diagnosis, Management, And Counseling In Newborns And Infants—Clinical Practice Guideline No. 6* (AHCPR pub. no. 93–0562). Rockville, MD: Agency for Health Care Policy and Research, Public Health Service, US Department of Health and Human Services, 1993.

Silverstein, A., V. B. Silverstein, and L. S. Nunn. *Sickle Cell Anemia*. Springfield, NJ: Enslow Publishers, Inc., 1997.

Simberkoff, M. S., A. P. Cross, M. Al-Ibrahim, A. L. Baltch, P. J. Geiseler, J. Nadler, A. S. Richmond, R. P. Smith, G. Schiffman, D. S. Shepard, J. P. Van Eeckhout. "Efficacy of pneumococcal vaccine in high-risk patients: Results of a Veteran Administration cooperative study." *New England Journal of Medicine* 315, no. 21 (1986): 1318–27.

Snyder, H. W., A. Mittelman, A. Oral, G. L. Messerschmidt, D. H. Henry, S. Korec, J. H. Bertran, T. H. Guthrie Jr., D. Ciarella, D. Wuest, W. Perkins, J. P. Balint Jr., S. K. Cochran, R. Pengout, and F. R. Jones. "Treatment of cancer chemotherapy-associated thrombotic thrombocytopenic/hemolytic uremic syndrome by protein A immunoadsorption of plasma." *Cancer* 71, no. 5 (1993):1882–92.

Solanki, D. L., G. G. Kletter, O. Castro. "Acute splenic sequestration crises in adults with sickle cell disease." *American Journal of Medicine* 80, no. 5 (1986): 985–90.

Solberg, C. O. "Meningococcal infections." In *Harrison's Principles of Internal Medicine, 14th ed.*, ed. A. S. Fauci, E. Braunwald, D. L. Kaspar, S. L. Hauser, D. L. Longo, J. L. Jameson, and J. Loscalzo, 910–15. New York: McGraw-Hill, 1998.

Solerte, S. B., and E. Ferrari. "Diabetic retinal vascular complications and erythrocyte filtrability: Results of a two-year follow-up study with pentoxifylline." *Pharmatherapeutica* 4, no. 6 (1985): 341–49.

Steinberg, M. H. "Management of sickle cell disease." *New England Journal of Medicine* 340, no. 13 (1999): 1021–30.

Steinberg, M. H., F. Barton, O. Castro, et al. "Effect of hydroxyurea on mortality and morbidity in adult sickle cell anemia: Risks and benefits up to 9 years of treatment." *Journal of the American Medical Association* 289, no. 13 (2003): 1645–51.

Steketee, R. W., J. J. Wirima, L. Slutsker, C. O. Khoromana, D. L. Heymann, and J. G. Breman. "Malaria treatment and prevention in pregnancy: The indications for use and adverse events associated with use of chloroquine and mefloquine." *American Journal of Tropical Medicine and Hygiene* 55, 1 suppl (1996): 50–56.

Stuart, M., R. Nagel. "Sickle cell disease." *Lancet* 364, no. 9442 (2004): 1343–60.

Styles, L. A., and E. Vichinsky. "Effects of a long-term transfusion regimen on sickle cell-related illnesses." *Journal of Pediatrics* 125, no. 6 pt. 1 (1994): 909–11.

Thomas, P. W., D. R. Higgs, and G. R. Serjeant. Benign clinical course in homozygous sickle cell disease: A search for predictors. *Journal of Clinical Epidemiology* 50, no. 2 (1997): 121–26.

Thompson, B. W., S. T. Miller, Z. R. Rogers, R. C. Rees, R. E. Ware, M. A. Waclawiw, R. V. Iyer, J. F. Casella, L. Luchtman-Jones, S. Rana, C. D. Thornburg, R. V. Kalpatthi, J. C. Barredo, R. C. Brown, S. Sarnaik, T. H. Howard, L. Luck and W. C. Wang. "The pediatric hydroxyurea phase III clinical trial (BABY HUG): Challenges of study design." *Pediatric Blood & Cancer* 54, no 2 (2010): 250-255.

Treacy, E., B. Childs, and C. R. Scriver. 1995. Response to treatment in hereditary metabolic disease. *American Journal of Human Genetics* 56(2):359–67.

University of Texas Health Science Center. 1995. Pathophysiology and management of sickle cell pain crisis: Report of a meeting of physicians and scientists, University of Texas Health Science Center at Houston, Texas. *Lancet* 346: 1408–11.

US Public Law 92-294. National sickle cell anemia control act of 1972. US Statutes at Large 86: 138.

Valle, D. "Treatment and prevention of genetic disease." In *Harrison's Principles of Internal Medicine, 14th ed.*, ed. A. S. Fauci, E. Braunwald, D. L. Kaspar, S. L. Hauser, D. L. Longo, J. L. Jameson, and J. Loscalzo, 403–09. New York: McGraw-Hill, 1998.

Vichinsky, E. P. "New therapies in sickle cell disease." *Lancet* 360, no. 9333 (2002): 629–31.

Vichinsky, E. P., C. M. Haberkern, L. D. Neumayr, et al. "A comparison of conservative and aggressive transfusion regimens in the perioperative management of sickle cell disease." *New England Journal of Medicine* 333, no. 4 (1995): 206–13.

Vichinsky, E. P., L. D. Neumayr, A. N. Earles, R. Williams, E. T. Lennette, D. Dean, B. Nickerson, E. Orringer, V. McKie, R. Bellevue, C. Daeschner, and E. A. Manci. "Causes and outcomes of the acute chest syndrome in sickle cell disease—National acute chest syndrome study group." *New England Journal of Medicine* 342, no. 25 (2000): 1855–65.

Vichinsky, E. P., O. Onyekwere, J. Porter, P. Swerdlow, et al. "A randomised comparison of deferasirox versus deferoxamine for the treatment of transfusional iron overload in sickle cell disease." *British Journal of Haematology* 136, no. 3 (2007): 501–08.

Wahl, S., and K. C. Quirolo. "Current issues in blood transfusion forsickle cell disease." *Current Opinion in Pediatrics* 21, no. 1 (2009): 15–21.

Walters, M. C., K. Ohene-Frempong, M. Patience, W. Leisenring, J. R. Eckman, J. P. Scott, W. C. Mentzer, S. C. Davies, F. Bernandin, D. C. Matthews, R. Storb, and K. M. Sullivan. "Bone marrow transplantation for sickle cell disease." *New England Journal of Medicine* 335, no. 6 (1996): 369–76.

Walters, M. C., M. Patience, W. Leisenring, et al. "Collaborative multicenter investigation of marrow transplantation for sickle cell disease: Current results and future directions." *Biology of Blood and Marrow Transplantation* 3, no. 6 (1997): 310–15.

Wang, W. C., R. W. Helms, H. S. Lynn, R. Redding-Lallinger, B. E. Gee, K. Ohene-Frempong, K. Smith-Whitley, M. A. Waclawiw, E. P. Vichinsky, L. A. Styles, R. E. Ware, and T. R. Kinney. "Effect of hydroxyurea on growth in children with sickle cell anemia: Results of the HUG-KIDS study." *Journal of Pediatrics* 140, no. 2 (2002): 225–29.

Ware, R. E. and R. W. Helms. "Stroke with transfusions changing to hydroxyurea (SWiTCH)." *Blood* 119 no. 17 (2012): 3925-3932.

Ware, R. E., W. H. Schultz, N. Yovetich, N. A. Mortier, O. Alvarez, L. Hilliard, R. V. Iyer, S. T. Miller, Z. R. Rogers, J. P. Scott, M. Waclawiw and R. W. Helms. "Stroke with transfusions changing to hydroxyurea (SWiTCH): a phase III randomized clinical trial for treatment of children with sickle cell anemia, stroke, and iron overload." *Pediatric Blood & Cancer* 57, no. 6 (2011): 1011-1017.

Wethers, D. L. "Sickle cell disease in childhood, part II: Diagnosis and treatment of major complications; Recent advances in treatment." *American Family Physicians* 62, no. 6 (2000): 1309–14.

Wikipedia, The Free Encyclopedia, s.v. "Introduction to Genetics," (accessed July 28, 2016), en.wikipedia.org/wiki/Introduction_to_genetics

Wison Schaeffer, J. J., K. M. Gil, M. Burchinal, K. D. Kramer, K. B. Nash, E. Orringer, and D. Strayhorn. "Depression, disease severity, and sickle cell disease." *Journal of Behavioral Medicine* 22, no. 2 (1999): 115–26.

Wun, T., T. Paglieroni, C. L. Field, J. Welborn, A. Cheung, N. J. Walker, and F. Tablin. "Platelet-erythrocyte adhesion in sickle cell disease." *Journal of Investigative Medicine* 47, no. 3 (1999): 121–27.

Xu, K., Z. M. Shi, L. L. Veeck, M. R. Hughes, and Z. Rosenwaks. "First unaffected pregnancy using preimplantation genetic diagnosis for sickle cell anemia." *Journal of the American Medical Association* 281, no. 18 (1999): 1701–06.

Yardley-Jones, A. "What are the implications of sickle cell anemia?" *Occupational Medicine (London)* 49, no. 1 (1999): 55–56.

Yawn, B. P., G. R. Buchanan, A. N. Afenyi-Annan et al. "Management of sickle cell disease: Summary of the 2014 evidence-based report by expert panel members." *Journal of the American Medical Association* 312, no. 10 (2014): 1033-1048.

Yoon, S. L., and A. Godwin. "Enhancing self-management in children with sickle cell disease through playing a CD-ROM educational game: A pilot study." *Pediatric Nursing* 33, no. 1 (2007): 60–63, 72.

Zimmerman, S. A., and R. E. Ware. "Palpable splenomegaly in children with hemoglobin SC disease: Hematological and clinical manifestations." *Clinical and Laboratory Haematology* 22, no. 3 (2000): 145–56.

Index

A

abdominal pain episodes, 14, 51, ,64, 138, 139, 165, 193
abortion, 206, 207, 209
acetaminophen, 45, 53, 64, 95, 134–135
acidosis, lactic, 20, 29, 51, 132
acute chest syndrome, 13, 15, 16, 19, 27, 50, 53, 59, 76, 96-97, 119, 121, 125, 127, 128, 143, 152, 156, 228, 234
acute sickle dactylitis, 13, 43
adoption, 93, 206
African Americans, 11, 12, 26, 78, 79, 97, 109, 153, 182, 190
AIDS, 72, 73
    HIV infection, 62, 72, 73, 74, 119, 121
air, 18, 19, 29–30, 87, 92
air travel, 19, 29–30
    and cabin pressure, 29
    and high altitudes, 18, 19, 26, 29, 87, 191, 194
alcohol, 18, 22, 70–71, 74, 79, 87, 132, 134
alloimmunization, 120
American Sickle Cell Anemia Association, 211
amino acids, 4, 7, 155, 198, 229
amniocentesis, 86, 203, 234
anemia, xi, 5, 6, 7, 8-9, 10, 11, 12, 13, 14, 15–16, 26, 27, 32, 33, 51–52, 56, 59, 61, 63, 79, 80, 83, 96, 97, 100, 113, 115, 152, 153, 154, 155, 158, 186, 191, 198, 199, 202, 207, 234
    aplastic, 16, 28, 52, 92, 234
    causes, 6, 234
    severe, 8, 51–52, 154
anesthesiologist, 107, 128
anti-anxiety medications, 151
antibiotics, 13, 17, 24, 52, 69, 96, 106, 126. *See also penicillin.*
antidepressants, 70, 98, 137–138, 148, 151
anxiety, 98–99, 106, 141, 145-146, 147, 151
appendicitis, 51, 133
arthritis medications, 81, 137
aspirin, 134–135, 136
asthma, 19, 87, 97, 105, 124, 134
auto-splenectomy, 51
avascular necrosis, 8, 9, 29, 59, 81–82, 84, 95, 105

B

balancing your soul, 149–150
bed wetting, 16, 56, 58
biliary colic, 14
bilirubin, 5, 8, 14, 44, 52, 56, 57, 63, 80, 115, 118
birth, 10, 26, 40, 43, 45, 52, 78, 122, 152
birth control, 71, 72–73
birth defects, 60–61, 84, 85, 153, 206, 207

blood, xi, xii, xiii, xiv, 2–6, 8, 9, 10, 12, 13, 14, 15–16, 17, 18, 22, 26, 28, 29, 32, 33, 41, 42, 43, 44, 45, 46, 47, 48–49, 50, 51, 52, 56, 57, 58, 60, 61, 62, 64, 69, 70-71, 72, 73, 76, 79, 80, 81, 82, 83, 84, 86, 87, 88, 92, 94, 96, 97, 98, 104, 105, 113, 115, 116, 117, 118, 119, 120, 121-122, 123, 124, 125, 126, 128, 131, 133, 138, 139, 140, 142, 143, 152, 153, 154, 155, 156, 158, 159, 161, 162, 163, 164, 166, 168, 169, 170, 183, 186, 191, 192, 194, 195, 196–197, 198, 199, 200, 201. *See also bone marrow, capillaries, hemoglobin, transfusions*
    cells (three types), 2–4
    chemistry values, 115, 139
    clots, 26, 72, 80, 97, 98, 125, 128, 142, 143, 192
    count, 41, 47, 61-62, 87, 115, 116, 119, 139, 143, 153, 154, 155, 191, 198, 235
    donating, 33, 64, 183
    drives, 33, 64, 183
    exchange transfusion, 96, 119, 120, 121, 122, 126, 128
    fluid overload, 120
    hepatitis B, 121
    HIV infection, 62, 72, 73, 74, 119, 121
    iron overload, 49, 85, 120, 121, 122, 123
    platelets, 2, 3–4, 5, 12, 59, 60, 115, 117, 134, 135, 153, 154, 163, 167
    red cells, xi, 2–3, 4, 5–6, 7, 9, 10, 12, 13, 15, 19, 21, 57, 58, 60, 63, 96, 97, 115, 118, 119, 120, 121, 122, 140, 152, 155, 167, 190, 191, 197, 198, 199, 200
    strokes, xi, xii, 8, 9, 13, 15, 16, 27, 28, 30, 33, 41, 48–50, 53, 56, 59, 61, 64, 67, 76, 99, 105, 119, 120, 121, 123, 125, 137, 142, 155, 158, 161, 164, 192, 196, 231, 237
    thickness, 120
    transfusions, xii, xiv, 8, 13, 16, 33, 34, 48–49, 50, 53, 57, 62, 64, 77, 79, 81, 83, 85, 92, 95, 96, 100, 118, 120-122, 123, 125, 126, 128, 129, 152, 153, 158, 159, 161, 163, 183, 200, 230-231, 232. *See also transfusions*
    vessels, xi, 2, 3, 4, 5, 7, 8, 12, 13, 16, 29, 32, 44, 48, 50, 51, 52, 57, 59, 70, 80, 82, 96, 97, 105, 124, 125, 126
    white cells, 2, 3, 4, 5, 12, 50, 59–60, 80, 115, 117, 119, 123, 153, 154, 163, 165, 167
blow bottle. *See incentive spirometer.*
bone infection, 14, 46, 69
    chronic, 69
bone marrow, xii, 4–5, 6, 8, 13, 27, 33, 44, 45, 49, 51, 52, 53, 56, 59, 62, 96, 97, 111, 113, 115, 131, 153, 158-166, 167, 168, 170, 171, 183, 203, 208, 231, 234
bone marrow transplants, xii, 4, 5, 27, 33, 49, 53, 62, 111, 113, 158-166, 167, 171, 183, 202, 208, 230, 232, 234
    complications, 53, 158, 159, 164-166
    cost, 111, 159
    future of, 166
    post-transplantation, 163
    preparing, 162
    risks of, 159
bone pain, 14, 51, 95, 100
bone scans, 69, 126
books, 37, 139, 219-222
BUN (blood urea nitrogen), 118

C

caffeine, 18, 19
camps, 24, 33, 55, 64, 109, 182, 183, 185
cancer screening, 98, 101
capillaries, 3, 5
career choices, 37, 73, 87, 88, 107
carrier, xiii, 7, 10, 11, 12, 83, 190, 191, 196, 198, 202, 204, 234
ceftriaxone, 24
chaplains, 106–107, 143
chelation, 122–123, 125

chest pain, 15, 19, 21, 50, 64, 96, 138, 139, 181
children, xi, xii, xiii, 8, 9, 13, 14, 16, 17, 18, 21, 22, 24, 26, 27, 28, 30, 31, 34–38, 40–76, 83, 84, 85, 86, 111, 114, 122, 125, 131, 135, 136, 152, 153, 159, 160, 171, 182, 185, 190, 191, 196
   healthy diet, 30–32
chorionic villus sampling, 86, 206, 207, 234
chromosome, 170, 197, 198, 234
ciprofloxacin, 24
climate, 28
clinical issues, 40–42, 54, 73, 87
clinical trials, 69-70, 173, 175–180
   informed consent, 162, 178
   phases, 177
   protocol, 176–177, 179
   types, 176-177
clots, 3–4, 26, 49, 72, 80, 97, 98, 125, 126, 128, 142, 143, 192, 196
   strokes, 49
codeine, 134, 135
complete blood count, 41, 87, 115, 139, 154, 155, 191, 198, 235
complications, 44–52, 57–58, 164–166, 192. *See also bone marrow transplants and trait.*
   prevention of, 194-195
constipation, 31, 83, 135, 137, 140, 143, 156
costs of care, 16–17, 37–38, 110–115, 122, 156, 159, 161, 180
   of bone marrow transplant, 53, 159
   of emergency room, 110
   of hospital stay, 110
CT, 48, 125
Cure Sickle Cell Initiative, 173, 233

D

dactylitis. *See hand-foot syndrome*
Demerol, 67, 140
depression, 16, 66, 70, 74, 99, 106, 138, 141, 143, 145–151, 186
   antidepressants, 70, 98, 137-138, 148, 151
chronic pain, 137, 138
   managing, 143, 147–151
dialysis, 96
diet, healthy, 30–32
disability law in schools, 64-65
DNA, 4, 5, 7, 9, 119, 167, 168, 169, 170, 171, 172, 173, 197, 202, 206, 207, 226, 228, 229, 231
doctors, 6, 17, 18, 19, 21, 30, 31, 32, 34, 41, 42, 46, 47, 48, 54, 55, 56, 60, 62, 67, 68, 75, 76, 77, 79, 80, 81, 82, 83, 84, 88, 95, 96, 98, 99, 104, 105, 106, 108, 109, 110, 112, 113, 114, 117, 125, 127, 128, 129, 132, 134, 135, 139, 143, 148, 151, 153, 156, 157, 158, 160, 161, 162, 164, 166, 167, 178, 180, 194, 204, 206, 208

E

emergency rooms, 105, 108, 109, 138. *See also hospital stay*
   cost of, 110
   pain relief, 135, 139–140
Endari, 155, 156-157, 233. *See also L-glutamine*
erection, painful. *See priapism*
erythropoietin, 6, 96, 100
eye examination, 9, 54, 83, 87, 104, 124–125
eye problems, 9, 82–83

F

family issues, 88, 99
family practitioner, 76, 112
fetal gamma gene, 170, 171
FARMS (memory device), 17-18, 55, 58, 70, 87, 98, 101, 235
ferritin, 118, 122, 123
fever, 13, 15, 17, 18, 19, 21, 27, 40, 44, 45, 46, 47, 50, 51, 53, 64, 65, 96, 119, 131, 132, 133, 134, 135, 138, 139, 193
fiber, importance of, 31, 83, 135
fluids, importance of, 18–19, 30
folic acid (folate), 8, 18, 21, 31–32, 41, 85, 87, 230

263

fundraising, 101, 181

G

gallbladder, 15, 51, 57, 80, 105, 143, 235
gallstones, 8, 14, 52, 54, 57, 80, 87, 118, 124, 142, 143, 236
genes, 8, 12, 35, 166, 168, 169, 170, 171, 172, 195, 197, 199, 227, 228, 231, 236
gene therapy, 86, 167-174, 207, 233, 236
genetic counseling, 10, 36, 73, 109, 195, 202-209
    preimplantation, 205, 207
genetic diseases, xi, xii, 168, 171, 173, 184, 197, 198, 202, 207, 226. *See also hemoglobinopathies, sickle cell disease, sickle cell trait, and thalassemias.*
genetics, 25, 83, 100, 196, 197-201, 202-209
Georgia Comprehensive Sickle Cell Center, xiii, 25, 110, 142
Grady Memorial Hospital. *See Georgia Comprehensive Sickle Cell Center*
graft rejection, 59, 164-165
graft-versus-host disease, 158, 159, 164
growth and development, 14, 15, 31, 35, 41, 55, 56, 57, 61, 70, 73, 75, 123, 152

H

hand-foot syndrome (dactylitis), 13, 15, 41, 43, 44-45, 236
health fairs, 109, 183
Health Maintenance Organizations. *See HMOs*
health passport, 225
hearing tests, 54, 123, 125
hematocrit, 115, 154
hematologist, 61, 76, 85, 104, 105, 108, 113, 117, 161, 191, 209
hemoglobin, xi, xii, 3, 4, 5, 6, 7, 8, 9, 10, 11, 12, 13, 14, 15, 19, 20, 26, 27, 36, 40, 43, 44, 46, 48, 51, 52, 56, 57, 60, 76, 77, 78, 82, 83, 85, 96, 101, 100, 115, 116, 118, 120, 121, 123, 128, 131, 152, 154, 164, 168, 169, 170, 171, 173, 174, 183, 190, 191, 192, 194, 195, 197-198, 199, 202, 203, 204, 208, 236
hemoglobin AS, 191, 236
hemoglobin C, 11, 26, 195, 198
hemoglobin E, 198, 199
hemoglobin electrophoresis, 10, 40, 78, 118, 164, 183, 191, 192, 198, 236
hemoglobin F, 10, 13, 152, 197
hemoglobin S beta thalassemia, 9, 10, 11, 51, 83, 170, 171, 190, 195, 198, 199, 203, 236
hemoglobin S-HPFH, 8, 10
hemoglobin SC, 9, 27, 191, 199, 236
hemoglobin SS. *See sickle cell anemia.*
hemoglobin SD-Punjab, 8
hemoglobin SE, 10, 199
hemoglobin SO-Arab, 8, 10, 199
hemoglobinopathies, 7, 46, 197, 202
hemolysis, xi, 6, 9, 56, 57, 97, 115, 236
hemophilia, 184, 227
hemophilus influenza, 23, 45
hip, avascular necrosis of, 8, 9, 29, 59, 81-82, 84, 105
human leukocyte antigen (HLA), 49, 53, 160, 161
HMOs, 38, 108, 111, 112-113
hospital stay, 110, 127-128, 142-143. *See also emergency rooms*
    admission, 142
    cost, 110
    in-patient care, 108, 110, 130, 143
    pain management, 131-132, 138-140, 142-143
hydrocodone, 134, 135
hydroxyurea, xi, xii, 10, 13, 18, 21, 27, 41, 53, 59-62, 70, 79, 84, 87, 95, 97, 100, 101, 110, 115, 117, 123, 156, 236
    alternatives, 62
    and birth defects, 60-61, 84, 153
    and hemoglobin F, 10, 152
    benefits, 59, 152-153
    cost, 110

monitoring, 60, 61
side effects, 59–60
hydroxyzine, 140, 151

I
ibuprofen, 64, 134, 135, 136, 140
immunizations, 17, 21, 22–24, 40, 41, 42, 45, 53, 73, 87, 111, 112, 115
  recommended, 23, 24, 31, 53
in vitro fertilization, 86, 207
incentive spirometer, 53, 82, 96, 127, 128, 143
infants. *See also* children, newborns
  birth–6 months, 40–41
  6 months–1 year, 41
infections, xi, 3, 4, 6, 8, 9, 12, 13, 14, 15, 16, 17, 21, 22, 23, 24, 27, 29, 31, 33, 41, 42, 44, 45–46, 49, 50, 51, 52, 53, 57, 60, 62, 63, 69, 72, 80, 82, 118, 119, 120, 121, 122, 125, 126, 132, 134, 139, 142, 154, 159, 163, 164, 165, 190, 198, 204
  blood tests, 119
influenza vaccine, 23, 45, 97
insurance. *See medical insurance*
internist, 76, 112
iron overload, 49, 85, 120, 121, 122, 123
  chelation therapy, 122–123
IV (intravenous) fluids, 16, 19, 50, 51, 119, 126, 236

J
jaundice, 8, 15, 44, 52, 56, 65, 164, 189, 193, 237

K
ketorolac, 140
kidney problems, 16, 51, 54, 58, 95–96, 105, 134, 164, 196

L
L-glutamine, xii, 155, 233. *See also* Endari
lab tests. *See tests*
lactose intolerance, 31, 153
LDH, 115

leg ulcers, 15, 70, 80–81, 88, 160
  treatment, 80–81
leukemia, 60, 154, 160, 171
life expectancy, xi, 9, 21, 25, 27, 63, 98, 186, 199
lung problems, 28, 51, 96–97, 105, 161

M
malaria, 12, 24–25, 26, 44, 190
mean corpuscular volume, 115, 198
Medicaid, 38, 111
medical attention, seeking, 14, 38, 53, 80, 87, 131, 146
medical care, 21–22, 104–129
  chaplains, 106–107, 143
  clinics, 108–110
  common procedures, 119–126
  costs, 110–115, 37–38
  doctors, 104–105
  emergency rooms, 109
  genetic counselors, 107–108
  medical insurance, 111–114
  nurses, 105–106
  physical therapists, 107
  psychiatrists, 106
  psychologists, 106
  sickle cell centers, 108–109
  social workers, 106
  tests, 115–119
medical insurance, 38, 111–114. *See also HMOs, Medicaid, Medicare, PPOs*
  options, 111
  fee-for-service plans, 113–114
medical procedures. *See also tests*
  bone scans, 69, 126
  chelation therapy, 122–123
  CT and MRI scans, 125
  eye examinations, 9, 54, 83, 87, 104, 124–125
  hearing tests, 54, 123, 125
  IV fluids, 16, 19, 50, 51, 119, 126, 127, 236
  pulmonary function, 54, 124
  skin test, 87
  transcranial Doppler (TCD), 13, 41, 49–50, 59, 125, 237
  transfusion therapy, 81, 118,

265

119-122
ultrasound, 49, 54, 59, 124, 125
X-rays, 50, 69, 105, 110, 119, 125
medical records, 129
medical tests. *See tests*
Medicare, 38, 114
medications, xi, xiv, 4, 14, 17, 18, 19, 21, 24, 27, 30, 31, 34, 57, 58, 60, 62, 70, 73, 75, 76, 80, 81, 82, 87, 95, 96, 99, 105, 106, 109, 110, 118, 119, 123, 126, 127, 128, 129, 133, 134, 135, 136, 137, 139, 140, 141, 142, 143, 148, 151, 153, 155, 156, 161, 165, 175, 176, 200, 201
   anti-anxiety, 151
   antidepressants, 70, 98, 137–138, 148, 151
   erythropoietin, 6, 96, 100
   hydroxyurea, xi, 10, 13, 18, 21, 27, 41, 53, 59–62, 70, 79, 84, 87, 95, 97, 100, 101, 110, 115, 123, 152–157, 236
   opiates, 31, 95, 96, 130, 134, 135, 137, 139-140, 141-142, 201
   pain, 14, 80, 96, 106, 127, 129, 133, 135, 136, 137, 139, 140, 201
   penicillin, 18, 21, 40, 41, 45, 52, 53, 54, 110, 160, 204, 230
Mendel, Gregor, 227-228
meningococcal vaccine, 23–24, 40
menopause, 97–98, 164
   bone mineral density test, 97
   hormone replacement therapy, 98
Meperidine, 140
morphine, 139–140
MRI, 48, 56, 111, 122, 125, 237

N

Nalbuphine, 140
National Institutes of Health, 27, 109, 130, 153, 155, 160, 173
National Marrow Donor Program, 160, 183
nephrologist, 105
newborns. *See also infants*
   penicillin, 52

and sickle cell screening, xi, 13, 27, 45, 184
nitric oxide, 32, 97
Noel, Walter Clement, 228
NSAIDs, 53, 83, 96, 134, 135, 136, 137
nurse practitioners, 105, 112, 127, 139
nurses, 42, 62, 75, 105–106, 108, 109, 110, 112, 127, 128, 129, 138, 143, 147, 178

O

obesity, 72
opiates, 95, 96, 130, 134, 135, 137, 140, 142, 201
   addiction to, 141–142
organ failure, 193
organizations, 109–110, 204, 211-218
orthopedic surgeon, 82, 105, 107
osteomyelitis. *See bone infection*
osteoporosis, 97–98

P

pain, xi, xiv, 7, 8, 9, 10, 12, 13, 14, 15, 16, 17, 18, 19, 20, 21, 22, 26, 27, 28, 29, 30, 31, 32, 33, 36, 37, 41, 42, 43, 44, 45, 50–51, 52, 53, 55, 57, 58, 59, 62, 63, 64, 66, 68, 69, 70, 71, 72, 76, 79–80, 81, 82, 84, 85, 87, 88, 94, 96, 97, 99, 100, 105, 106, 107, 109, 119, 120, 121, 127, 128, 129, 130–144, 145, 146, 147, 148, 149, 151, 152, 156, 157, 160, 161, 163, 165, 181, 182, 186, 191, 192, 193, 194, 198, 201
   causes of, 131
   chronic, 95, 99, 107, 130–131, 133, 135, 137–138, 141, 145, 146, 147, 148, 149, 151
   emergency rooms and, 138-141
   management, 130–144
   medications, 134-138, 139–141. *See also NSAIDs*
   patient-controlled analgesia pump, 127, 139, 140, 143
   recording, 132–133
   relaxation techniques, 143–144

treatment, 134–138
types of, 133–134
pain crises, 27, 28, 29, 50–51, 95, 100, 237. *See also pain*
triggers for, 20, 22, 28, 29, 51, 131
pain specialists, 105
parenting children with sickle cell disease, 34–38
child acting out, 42–43
financing medical care, 37–38
guilt, 35-36
requirements, 34–35
sick role, 55
support, 36
patient-controlled analgesia pump, 127, 139, 140, 143
pediatrician, 19, 104, 112, 206, 225
peer support, 73, 89, 99, 101
penicillin, 18, 21, 40, 41, 45, 52, 53, 54, 110, 160, 204, 230
newborns and, 40, 45, 52
physical issues, 15–16
physical therapists, 82, 107
physician assistants, 105, 127, 139
plasma, 2
platelets, 3–4, 5, 12, 59–60, 115, 134, 135, 153, 154, 163, 167, 234
pneumococcal vaccine, 21, 23, 40, 41
PPOs, 113
pregnancy, 83–86. *See also abortion, birth defects, in vitro fertilization, genetic counseling, preimplantation genetic diagnosis.*
avoiding, 205-206
preimplantation genetic diagnosis, 205, 207
priapism, 15, 16, 22, 57–58, 59, 69-70, 84, 105, 119, 142, 153, 237
psychiatrists and psychologists, 106
psychosocial issues, 16, 42–43, 54–55, 73–76, 87–88, 98–99, 101, 147
puberty, delayed, 15, 16, 33, 55, 57, 63, 70, 71, 74, 97
public, educating the, 33, 64, 183, 184
pulmonary function tests, 54, 124
pulmonary hypertension, 16, 70, 97, 122, 124, 237

R
red blood cells, xi, 2–3, 5, 6, 8, 9, 10, 12, 13, 14, 16, 18, 19, 31, 33, 44, 46, 47, 48, 51, 52, 53, 56, 57, 59, 60, 62, 70, 80, 81, 87, 96, 97, 115, 116, 117, 118, 119, 120, 121, 122, 124, 127, 129, 131, 133, 138, 139, 152, 153, 154, 156, 159, 163, 167, 168, 190, 197, 198, 199, 200
cycle of, 5–6
relaxation techniques, 143–144
research. *See treatments and research*
resources
books and booklets, 219-223
CD-ROMs, 213
clinics, 226
conferences and meetings, 223-224
National Marrow Donor Program, 160, 183
organizations, 211-218
scholarships, 225
sickle cell centers, 108-109, 225
Sickle Cell Disease Association of America, 110, 215
Sickle Cell Information Center, 32, 144, 211, 212, 219
smartphone apps, 226-227
videos, 218
websites, 211-214
reticulocytes, 5, 41, 87, 115, 116, 117, 139, 237
rifampin, 23

S
Salmonella, 46
scholarships, 109, 182, 185, 226
schools, 16, 24, 32–33, 34, 35, 42, 43, 54, 55, 56, 62–66, 70, 88, 106, 125, 186
and disabled children, 64-65
sickle cell classroom guide, 62–64
parental involvement, 65–66
sequestration, 8, 9, 13, 14, 15, 26, 41, 46-48, 52, 56, 76, 119, 120, 237. *See also spleen*
severe combined immune deficiency, 171

sexuality and teenagers, 71–73
sickle beta thalassemia, 9–10, 199
sickle C, 11, 26, 195, 198. *See also sickle cell trait*
sickle cell anemia (Hemoglobin SS), 7, 8, 9, 10, 11, 13, 14, 26, 27, 76, 79, 80, 83, 85, 97, 100, 115, 152, 153, 155, 158, 198, 199, 202, 207, 236
    symptoms of, 8
sickle cell centers, 78, 108–109
sickle cell disease (SCD)
    carriers, 7, 10, 190-196, 202, 234. *See also sickle cell trait*
    caused by, 7
    climate and, 28
    distribution, 11, 12
    guide for teachers and employers, 32–33, 62–66
    history, 226-233
    incidence in black populations, 11
    incidence in the United States, 11
    infections, 17
    life expectancy, 9, 21, 25
    myths, 25-28
    symptoms, 15–16
Sickle Cell Disease Association of America (SCDAA), 110, 215
sickle cell foundations, 33, 55, 64, 78, 109–110
Sickle Cell Information Center, 32, 144, 211, 212-213. *See also Georgia Comprehensive Sickle Cell Center*
sickle cell trait, 7, 11, 24, 26–27, 73, 83, 157, 159, 190-196, 198, 199, 203, 208, 236
    African Americans and, 190
    blood in urine, 26, 192, 194
    complications, 192-194
    genetic counseling, 202-209
    genetics and, 197
    hemoglobin C, 11, 26, 195
    incidence rate in African Americans, 190
    malaria, 12, 24–25, 190
    misdiagnoses, 191-192
skin test, 87

sleep, adequate, 20-21. *See also rest*
smoking, 19, 70, 87
social workers, 37, 38, 75, 76, 99, 106, 108, 111–112, 114, 115, 143, 161, 178
spleen, xi, 2, 3, 8, 9, 10, 13, 15, 17, 23, 29, 40, 41, 45, 46–47, 48, 51, 52, 56, 59, 105, 115, 124, 139, 193, 196, 237
    auto-splenectomy, 51
    enlarged, 9, 29, 47
    sequestration episode, 52
splenic sequestration, 8, 9, 13, 14, 15, 26, 41, 46-48, 52, 56, 76, 119, 120, 237
sports. *See also exercise*
    complications from, 29
    recommended, 28
    sprains and strains, 29
stem cell transplant, xii, 5, 27, 111, 169, 170, 171, 172. *See also bone marrow transplants*
stress, 13, 18, 21, 22, 29, 51, 58, 74, 99, 106, 131, 132, 145, 146, 186
strokes, xi, xii, 8, 9, 13, 15, 16, 27, 28, 30, 33, 41, 48–50, 53, 56, 59, 61, 64, 66, 76, 98, 105, 119, 120, 121, 123, 125, 137, 142, 155, 158, 161, 164, 196, 237
    prevention, 13, 49–50
    silent, 49
    symptoms, 48
    treatment, 49
sudden death, 192, 193, 196
summer camps, 33, 55, 56, 109, 182, 185
support groups, 18, 41, 43, 58, 73, 89, 109, 148, 186, 223-224
    peer, 73, 89, 99, 101
surgeons, 82, 105, 107
surgery, 9, 48, 58, 69, 80, 82, 83, 105, 107, 119, 128–129, 176
swimming, 18, 22, 28, 58
symptoms
    of sickle cell disease, 8, 15–16
    of stroke, 48

Index

T

TCD. *See transcranial Doppler ultrasound screening*
teacher guide, 32–33, 62–64
teenagers, 67–76. *See also young adults*
   birth control and, 72–73
   clinical issues, 73
   delayed puberty, 70, 74
   emotional problems, 70
   psychosocial issues, 73–74
   transition to adult care, 74–76
tests. *See also medical procedures*
   amniocentesis, 86, 206, 234
   blood chemistry, 115, 117
   bone scans, 69, 126
   BUN (blood urea nitrogen), 118
   chorionic villus sampling, 86, 206, 207, 235
   complete blood count, 41, 87, 115, 116-117, 139, 154, 155, 191, 198, 235
   creatinine, 118
   ferritin, 118, 122
   hemoglobin electrophoresis, 10, 40, 78, 118, 164, 183, 191, 192, 198, 236
   human leukocyte antigen (HLA), 159, 161
   infections, 69
   MRI, 48, 56, 111, 122, 125, 236
   platelet count, 117
   screening, 73
   urinary, 87, 118
   X-rays, 12, 26, 27, 31, 125
thalassemias, 7, 9–10, 11, 13, 49, 51, 59, 61, 79, 81, 82, 83, 115, 124, 152, 155, 170, 171, 190, 191, 195, 198, 199, 203
   alpha, 198, 199
   beta, 9–10, 198, 199, 203, 236
transcranial Doppler ultrasound screening, 13, 41, 49–50, 59, 125, 237
   and stroke prevention, 49–50, 125
transient ischemic attack, 48-49
travel precautions, 23, 24, 29–30, 194. *See also air travel*
treatments and research (new), 173-174
   clinical trials, 176-180
   gene therapy, 167-174
   hydroxyurea and glutamine, 152–157
   stem cell transplant, xii, 4–5, 27, 169, 170, 171, 172

V

vaccination. *See immunizations*
valine, 4, 198
videos, 37, 150, 218
vocational rehabilitation, 76, 107, 184

W

water, 18, 19, 20, 21, 28, 30, 31, 32, 33, 36, 58, 63, 83, 87, 97, 134, 135, 156, 192, 193, 194. *See also fluids*
weather, 22, 36, 46, 88
websites, 208–215. *See also resources*
white blood cells, 3, 12, 50, 59, 60, 80, 115, 119, 123, 153, 154, 163, 165

X

X-rays, 50, 69, 105, 110, 119, 125

Y

young adults, 77–89
   career choices, 88
   clinical issues, 87
   family issues, 88
   peer support, 89
   psychosocial issues, 87–88